DEMON IN MY BLOOD

# DEMON

## *IN MY*

# BLOOD

## My Fight with Hep C—
## and a Miracle Cure

ELIZABETH RAINS

GREYSTONE BOOKS
*Vancouver/Berkeley*

*To everyone who has ever been infected with hepatitis C,
and to Al for his patience and love throughout my illness*

Greystone Books Ltd.
www.greystonebooks.com

Cataloguing data available from Library and Archives Canada
ISBN 978-1-77164-170-8 (pbk.)
ISBN 978-1-77164-171-5 (epub)

Editing by Nancy Flight
Copyediting by Stephanie Fysh
Cover design by Peter Cocking
Text design by Nayeli Jimenez
Printed and bound in Canada on ancient-forest-friendly paper by Friesens

We gratefully acknowledge the support of the Canada Council for the
Arts, the British Columbia Arts Council, the Province of British Columbia
through the Book Publishing Tax Credit, and the Government of Canada
for our publishing activities.

Canadä

BRITISH
COLUMBIA  | BRITISH COLUMBIA
ARTS COUNCIL
An agency of the Province of British Columbia

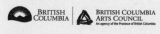

Canada Council   Conseil des arts
for the Arts     du Canada

# CONTENTS

# INTRODUCTION

WHEN MY DOCTOR said, "You have hepatitis C," it felt as if I had been propelled onto another planet. It was a desolate place with no landmarks.

I told my husband about the diagnosis, but no one else. Two days later a friend visited my home. Sitting on the beach with her, talking about her teaching project and about the best ways to moor a boat, I gave her less than half my attention. The rest of my mind tumbled in outer space. I thought about my disease all the time.

I was a journalist, so I immersed myself in research. I reasoned that by doing what I habitually do, I could stay objective and calm my fears about my illness. I read everything I could about hepatitis C and talked with everyone I could find who was an expert on the disease.

Eventually I contacted a publisher who wanted my story. My research continued for more than a year after that, past those early, fearful days, throughout my treatment, and beyond. The treatment, with direct-acting antivirals, was quick. The side effects were next to nothing. I was among the very first patients who were prescribed a groundbreaking non-interferon drug combination without participating in a clinical trial. My only big problem was the cost of the drug—close to $120,000 for the twelve-week regimen. But it worked. I am now 100 percent free of hepatitis C.

While writing this book, I met dedicated researchers who vowed to eradicate hep C from the earth, and I met dozens of people who suffer or have suffered from the illness. Most of the people with hepatitis C were baby boomers, past IV drug users, or both. Without exception, I found the researchers to be sincere about helping patients and about creating a future free from hepatitis C. I found the people who had contracted hep C to be philosophical and often charming and funny.

After the initial jolt of diagnosis, I first turned only to my husband and daughters for support. After a few weeks I began telling close friends about my disease. Most of them listened patiently as I expressed my fears about hepatitis C. They gave me comfort when I desperately needed it, and I will feel bound to these friends forever. But not all of my friends gave me comfort. Several showed prejudice about the disease or just didn't want to hear about it. Between my diagnosis and when I was declared disease free, I learned that some friends are friends from the deepness of their heart and others are friends from the surface of their mind. I didn't fault the surface friends, but I no longer felt close to them. I stopped talking with two of them entirely.

I also learned about greed. Principals at drug companies had set astounding prices on the latest hep C drugs. In addition to the simeprevir-sofosbuvir drug combination I took, many other easy hepatitis C treatments have emerged. Today, patients can take one pill a day instead of two, sometimes for fewer than twelve weeks. Still, the cost of treatment is more than most patients' yearly income. Insurance plans in the U.S. and provincial drug plans in Canada continue to refuse payment to many patients. Prices close to $1,000 per pill have generated scads of negative publicity for the drug companies, which have reacted by playing shy with journalists. I got around this as best I could and connected with a few key people in the companies. They provided valuable background information.

Some people I interviewed who have been afflicted with hepatitis C asked that their names be withheld. I have honored their requests by using pseudonyms. In some instances, I have altered other identifying information. I have stuck as close to reality as possible while aiming to respect people's wishes. Other sources' identities have been withheld for personal reasons.

I talked with people and looked at research from all over the world. However, most of my sources are based either near Vancouver, British Columbia, or in San Francisco. Vancouver is a typical Canadian city when it comes to hepatitis C treatment, and has been home to many clinical trials of hepatitis drugs. I live close to Vancouver and underwent treatment there. San Francisco, however, is not a typical American city in its approach to hepatitis C but a progressive city that is arguably home to North America's best support network for people seeking hep C treatment or counseling. When I asked for help in researching this book, hepatitis C patient advocates in San Francisco poured out an enormous welcome and led me to a wealth of resources. As a result, a large portion of the information in this book is from San Francisco.

When I first talked with my publisher, he encouraged me to dig deep into my hippie days, when I most likely contracted hepatitis C. He asked me to bring out the flavor of the sex, drugs, and rock 'n' roll era. I tried to reconstruct some of that past in this book to show ways I may have acquired hepatitis C. Some incidents include quotations. Most of the words were uttered so long ago that I have probably not repeated them accurately. However, I'm certain the words I've chosen reflect the speakers' intentions and meanings. I have aimed to characterize people and to explain their actions and emotions, which I remember well.

I've written about family incidents from my childhood and talked with my older sisters Mary and Kathy to check for accuracy. Each of us recalls events differently. I am much younger than they are, so the events I refer to were probably more traumatic for me. While I was considering our different viewpoints, I talked with John Lavette, a San Franciscan whose story is in this book. He described a scene with his father that was so disturbing to him, "it became like a photograph." The traumatic scenes from my own childhood were etched in my memory too. When all was said and done, I decided to go with my own version of childhood events, modified somewhat by my sisters' recollections.

I have blended these long-past experiences with my thoughts during treatment, with stories of other people who have hep, and with recent events surrounding hepatitis C. Coming through the disease, through the shock of the diagnosis, through the pain of learning of its stigma, through the relief of knowing I had people to support me, and through the insight I gained from meeting people who had bravely fought their own infection, I made some unexpected discoveries. I learned about friendship, medical science, and greed—and I learned that throughout my experience with hepatitis C, I was incredibly lucky.

By 2017, more than two years after the end of my treatment, the traditional hepatitis C remedy, six months to a year of grueling interferon, had diminished to a blip on the medical landscape. New drugs had turned treatment into a simple two or three months of easy pill-taking. Governments, health organizations, and at least one multinational drug manufacturer announced plans to eliminate the virus entirely.[1] Yet most people with hepatitis C still find it daunting to pay for the miracle drugs.

Thankfully, market forces have begun to shift, making hepatitis C treatment more affordable. I believe there is hope that one day this disease will be eradicated.

# DECEMBER 1971

A FLUFF OF CLOUD parted and sun danced through the windows as I entered the downtown Montreal apartment with my beautiful tiny baby. The four-room suite took up the whole second floor of the landlord's house. Peter, Della, and I had just moved in. The floors creaked and white paint was peeling from the wainscoting, but there was ample space for a soapstone-carving corner and for four-year-old Della to run around. Unlike Peter, I had wanted a second girl. My new child was unexpectedly fair, with pink cheeks and fine, wispy hair that was almost white. She gurgled in my arms. We would name her Jessica. I was reading *Dune,* and Jessica was the wise woman in the story.

Because I was young, healthy, and strong, I didn't let the doctor's order to get some rest stop me from playing with my four-year-old. I believed she needed assurance that I'd love her the same as always, even though I couldn't help grinning at the cute little honey bunny I had just brought home. I sat on the floor with Della, rolled out huge sheets of parchment, and opened a dozen jars of poster paint. Together we painted sheet after sheet of grassy fields that burst with flowers. We painted happy faces on suns that shone above the fields. When Della grew tired and curled into a nap, I made a mobile of ribbons, which I hung over Jessica's crib. I woke Jessica to feed and diaper her—she was, at first, a sleepy baby—and then fatigue dusted over me.

I awoke an hour or so later when I heard a knock. Peter answered the door and greeted Norman, a friend who was an intern at the Jewish General Hospital, where Jessica had been born. He had come to congratulate the new parents and to see the baby. As I was about to get up to say hello, I noticed that a blizzard was blowing outside and the mattress on the floor that served as my bed was soaked red with blood.

Norman saw what was happening and rolled his palms over my belly, trying to push out pieces of placenta so that the hemorrhage would stop. We used up all of my Kotex pads to sop up the flow, and then all of the baby diapers. But the red, sticky stream didn't abate. Norman carried me down the stairs to the snow-covered sidewalk and into his car. I remember the little beater Datsun swerving and screeching through icy streets. I remember snow blowing against the windscreen faster than the wipers could wipe. After that I passed out.

I awoke for a minute or two in the hospital emergency room. A nurse said I had lost so much blood that she couldn't find my pulse. Needles attached to tubes stuck out of my arms, and one was flowing crimson. I passed out again, unaware that the demon that would threaten my life forty years later had most likely just sloshed into my veins.

# PART I

*INFESTATION*

## CHAPTER 1

# FATIGUE

SALT WATER SPLASHED my face and soaked my shirt. It lapped at my feet in the bottom of the sleek sea kayak. My hands gripped the paddle, plunging it in and out of the surf, but not fast enough. Not hard enough. Waves knocked the side of the kayak, threatening to swamp me. A cedar home on the bluff above the rocky beach to my right, which I had admired ten minutes earlier, was still directly to my right. The kayak bobbed and pitched, but I was making no headway against the current.

I struggled to will away the fatigue that had plagued me lately, but I couldn't find the energy to coax the boat even a foot forward through the sea. Wind blew at me. I was so, so tired. I worked the rudder but couldn't make the boat turn toward shore. I thought the kayak would fill with water and I would drown.

I was on a visit to Mayne Island, in British Columbia, with two of my colleagues at the college where I taught. We knew that the currents between Lizard and Samuel islands would become turbulent around noon, so we had planned to glide through the passage by eleven. But we had lingered over coffee and had stopped a few times to take pictures.

An hour into the paddling trip, my friends Cheryl and Abbe had become used to my pausing for rest and camera shots, and we had set a pattern of one or both of them cruising ahead and waiting. Just after we had turned into the passage, they advanced out of sight. They were probably far ahead, past the rough stretch, waiting for me. They could wait forever, it seemed, and I would never catch up with them. I realized that if the boat were to capsize, I would stay conscious only for a while. I was too tired to paddle, so certainly I was also too tired to swim. Too bad I had never learned the kayak roll. Too bad that somehow the strength I used to possess had ebbed.

I stopped paddling to see where the current would take me and also because I could hardly move my body anymore. I couldn't catch my breath. A wave breached the rail and spat into my mouth as I was yawning.

I had always been muscular for a woman and believed I had retained above-average stamina. During my thirties I had lifted weights in a gym about ten hours a week. During my forties I had been a yoga fanatic. But now, in my fifties, I became easily exhausted. I felt generally weak and would give up on household chores after half an hour because of a desperate need for a nap. Maybe the fatigue was a normal consequence of getting older, I thought.

Just as I was about to let the sea take me wherever it would, I saw red hair gleaming in the sun. It was Cheryl in her kayak, plowing through the surf. She roped my kayak to hers and towed me until we were near the shore. Then I paddled sluggishly alongside her to Potato Point on Mayne Island, where Abbe waited, smiling and cheering me in.

Cheryl and Abbe were close to my age, and they had plenty of energy. What was the matter with me?

After that experience, I decided that the problem was that I was overworked. I had two jobs, too many students, and little time to spare. Retirement would cure me, I was sure. To prepare for it and for our dream life of ease, in the late summer of 2012 my husband and I moved away from Vancouver into an ocean-view home on forested land on the Sunshine Coast of British Columbia. My plan was to work there for a few more years and then to enjoy my family and travel.

The Sunshine Coast is a peninsula, lying twelve miles from Greater Vancouver across Howe Sound. A ridge of the Coast Mountains surrounds the sound, creating eye-popping seascapes but making road travel to Vancouver impossible. To get from the rural coast to Vancouver's frantic metropolis, we had to take a ferry. Al and I both worked there. We commuted two hours each way—on the boat, bus, and SkyTrain—for our jobs.

Leaving at 5:45 a.m. to catch the ferry was tough because I rarely got enough sleep. Besides being tired in the day, I suffered joint pain in my arm and shoulder at night. I was also unusually jittery. No matter when I got to bed, a stabbing pain would jar me awake close to midnight. The only relief was to sit upright for at least an hour. I kept both a Kindle and an Android reader on my bedside table, each loaded with several books. I would fire one up, place three pillows behind my back, and read. Eventually I would flop into sleep, but I would suffer a couple more bouts of anguish before dawn. The routine often woke my husband. Al, ever tolerant and an easy sleeper, would half open his eyes and ask what was wrong. I remember a night when I answered by snapping, "Don't you know?" I tossed the Kindle aside and knocked my lamp onto the floor, shattering its bulb. I had thought living on the quiet Sunshine Coast would keep me relaxed, but it didn't.

Soon after the move, I learned that my doctor in Vancouver was thinking of retiring. After thirty years of a doctor–patient relationship, Dr. Louise Halliman and I had become friends. I told her I planned to retire soon too. So as Louise tested my damaged arm for mobility, we talked about opening up time in our lives during retirement. It seemed the right time to try a doctor on my side of the ferry route.

Back at home I called Dr. Iris Radev, who had just begun to practice in Gibsons. Her assistant slotted me into a "meet and greet" appointment for March 10, 2014. As the day approached, I decided I'd interview Dr. Radev, find out if I liked her manner, and withhold my decision whether to change doctors until I had given it some thought. Dr. Radev turned out to be a perky young woman in a trendy gray business suit. Perched at a computer, she tapped away as she asked about my medical history. She started with the usual set of questions: Any history of cancer in my family? Heart problems? Major surgery? No, no, no. The questions kept coming—there were more than I was used to—and she mentioned that she liked to be thorough. She examined my heartbeat with a stethoscope, and she looked down my throat with a tongue depressor. She asked about my medications, and she filled out a prescription for one that was running low. She typed the information into the computer with fingers almost blurry with speed. A printer churned out the prescription. I gazed on in appreciation, my plans to treat the "meet and greet" like a job interview as far out the window as China is from my living room.

The printer kept spitting out pages. "These are for tests," she said, handing me some of the sheets. "When I get a new patient, I do a lot of tests."

I thanked my new doctor and headed out of the clinic into the sunlit parking lot. Unlike medical labs in Vancouver and its suburbs, the LifeLabs unit in Gibsons is seldom busy. In fact, a ten-minute wait for anything on the Sunshine Coast except the ferry is considered exceedingly long. So as I walked out of the Gibsons Medical Clinic I had no excuse not to pop into LifeLabs. The sun shone. Spring was coming, and potted pansies bloomed on racks outside the grocery store. Ambling through the parking lot, I glanced through the lab's sidewalk-to-ceiling windows. The waiting room was empty. I gazed at the top sheet in my hand and read that one of the tests would be a blood test. I turned and walked straight to my car. After all, my dog, Zeena, was alone at home, wanting a walk. I told myself the tests were routine. There was no urgency.

Actually, I knew Zeena could wait. I was skittish around anything that could draw blood. I had fainted twice during blood tests, and once in the 1980s I wobbled with my stomach churning as a doctor sliced a quarter-inch sample of a rash from my young daughter's shoulder. Both Jessica and the doctor reached out to steady me, and I squirmed in embarrassment. The incident reinforced my squeamishness, which prompted me to sidestep Dr. Radev's order for a blood test.

Besides asking me to get the blood test, Dr. Radev had recommended that I see a physiotherapist for my joint pain. The physiotherapist wanted a copy of MRI results from tests that had been done on my shoulder the year before. Close to two weeks after my first visit with Dr. Radev, I stopped at the clinic to ask for those. Since I'd be in the same mall,

I decided to go to LifeLabs. As I left the medical clinic, I conveniently skipped the second task and drove instead to Tim Hortons.

Driving home with a coffee in the cup holder and a honey cruller in hand, I scolded myself for being a wimp. My husband and I would be leaving the next month for Mexico. Before splashing into the ocean off Tulum, I should make sure I was healthy. So I got off the main drag, made a U-ey, and drove through Upper Gibsons to the mall. My fingers were sticky from the donut, so I took a side trip to a washroom at the nearby supermarket. I continued on to the medical lab, stopping at a clothing store to try on some jeans and at a kitchen store to hunt for a cheese grater. I wandered through the Sears outlet store, comparing major appliances I didn't need. Then I steeled myself and entered LifeLabs.

The waiting room was empty. I started to leave, but a short, curly-haired lab assistant named Bernice arrived at the counter and reached for my requisition. Once I handed it to her I was committed.

"You can go right ahead," Bernice said. She led me to a room with a beige padded chair fitted with wide, beige padded arms that went well with the beige-everything look of the clinic.

"I can't sit. I'll faint," I said, thinking my blood would create a startling contrast with the decor.

Bernice led me to another room with a narrow vinyl bed that had a sterile paper cloth spanning its length. I lay down, stretched out my arm, and squinted my eyes shut. I explained I had fainted in the past.

"Don't worry," she said. "It won't take long. You can stay here and lie down afterward, until you feel okay." She babbled about the weather and stretched a tourniquet around my arm. A needle pierced my skin. Seconds slushed by. My stomach fell, as if I were descending in a roller coaster. "All done," she said.

My mind spun for a few minutes, and then I slowly rose from the cot. As I passed Bernice at the counter, I grabbed a brochure that told me I could get my results online. I was happy I hadn't fainted. (It's hard to swoon while lying down.) I could get the results quickly. And I wouldn't need another blood test anytime soon, I told myself, unless the test revealed I had hemochromatosis.

HEMOCHROMATOSIS IS A rare genetic disease that causes a dangerous iron overload in the blood. It affects more than 1 million Americans and 100,000 Canadians. It's most common among people of northern European descent. Its symptoms include abdominal pain and memory fog, which I had been experiencing. I knew the source of my stomach pain. It was a hiatal hernia, in which stomach acid flushes upward through the diaphragm and flows where it shouldn't. I attributed the memory fog—which I later learned is also a symptom of hep—to a loss of sleep because of shoulder pain. However, my dad had suffered from hemochromatosis, so he carried the gene. He had advised me to get tested. For many years I had put his warning aside.

It had come a few weeks before he died, and less than a month after 9/11. The highway borders between British Columbia and Seattle had thickened with security. Lineups for cars were inordinately long, and most people avoided cross-border trips. I couldn't do that. My dad was suffering from heart disease, bone cancer, and kidney failure. My mother was having a hard time managing the half-hour drive from their condo in Kent to downtown Seattle to take my dad to his dialysis appointments. I crossed the border once or twice a week to help out.

After driving forty minutes from Vancouver, I'd line up with hundreds of other frustrated drivers and wait. Eventually I'd inch up to the Customs and Immigration window, hold out my passport, and explain I would be visiting my parents. I'd drive another three hours to Kent, which was halfway between Seattle and Tacoma. I would head out from Vancouver in the middle of the day and by the time I arrived in Seattle, I'd be caught in the rush hour. I was working at two jobs (and had hepatitis C without knowing it), so I would be tired, exasperated, and not in the mood to hear any of the invective my dad typically spewed whenever my mother or I said or did anything that wasn't entirely to his liking.

One day, while I was driving my parents to the kidney dialysis center, traffic became unusually heavy. I took a left turn at a busy intersection, where I knew of a shortcut. My dad snapped, "That's the wrong way."

"This is a shortcut. It will get us there," I said.

"You're an idiot. You don't know your way around Seattle."

"I've driven through here many times. Check the map. This is the right way, and it's quicker," I said, fumbling in the glove compartment and pulling out a map.

He refused to take it. "You're wrong. You're an idiot," he said.

"Maybe there's more than one route," my mother said from the back seat.

"You don't know anything, Julia. You're stupid and you've always been stupid. Now shut up," he boomed at her.

I pulled the car to the side of the busy road, onto a gravel driveway. "*You* shut up and apologize to Mother," I said.

"I'm not going to apologize. Turn around. Do what I say! Go back the way I told you."

"This is the right way, and I'm not going anywhere until you apologize to Mother."

My dad's rage rose toward the boiling point. He called me names much worse than "idiot." He called my mother "mindless" and "useless."

His rant continued for a minute or two, but it seemed to last an hour amid the hum of cars at the intersection. My hands tensed on the steering wheel, but I said nothing until he had stopped. "You're an old man," I said. "I assume you need to go to your dialysis appointment or you'll die sooner than you thought. But I'm not going anywhere until you apologize to Mother. You've abused her too much over the years. Now apologize."

He said nothing.

My mother said nothing.

"I'm not going anywhere," I said. Traffic whizzed by. I looked at my watch. It was a late-afternoon appointment and the dialysis center would soon close.

"I'm not an evil man," my father said.

"Then apologize."

"I apologize," he said.

"You apologize to Mother?"

"I apologize to Mother."

He spoke gruffly, without a sorry tone, but I had freaked myself out wondering if my stalling would kill him. I drove on. The shortcut worked. We reached the dialysis center on time.

My father didn't talk to me again that whole weekend, but the next time I arrived for a drive to the dialysis center, he pulled me aside and said, "There's something I've got to tell you. You should be tested for hemochromatosis."

He explained that it was a genetic disease. If my mother had a gene for it—she had never been tested—I would have a 50 percent chance of inheriting the illness. Hemochromatosis inhibits the elimination of iron from the blood. It causes excess iron to collect in the organs, including the heart, the kidneys, and the liver, and can make them fail.

ONE WEEK AFTER the blood test, I was sipping a morning coffee and reading the news on my tablet when I received a phone call from a medical assistant in Dr. Radev's office saying that Dr. Radev wanted me to come in. After I made an appointment, I turned to my computer and looked at My Ehealth, British Columbia's and Ontario's online system that provides lab results to patients. The site showed that my hematocrit and hemoglobin levels were beyond the normal range. Hematocrit is the percentage of red blood cells in the blood. Every red blood cell contains 280 million molecules of hemoglobin. Each molecule of hemoglobin contains four proteins of heme, an iron-based pigment that picks up, carries, and releases oxygen. Excess iron is the problem in hemochromatosis, so I figured that with too many red blood cells, hemoglobin, and iron-carrying proteins, I was a sure candidate for the disease.

The treatment for hemochromatosis, which my dad had begun too late to save his organs, is frequent phlebotomy, or removal of blood from the body with a syringe. I knew I had automatically inherited one of my dad's two hemochromatosis genes, and now I thought I must have picked up a recessive gene from my mother. I believed I would be subject to the most awful treatment I could imagine and would have to endure it for the rest of my life.

1953

# CHILD

THERE IS A small chance that I contracted hepatitis C when I was four. My parents had just bought a green stucco house in Bayside Gables, couched on the eastern edge of Queens where Long Island juts into the Atlantic. The Gables was nothing like what most people might imagine as New York City. The eight-block cluster of high-end homes adjoined a swamp, a mud-bottomed bay, and undeveloped forest. Most of our neighbors' homes hid behind scrolled-iron gateways or rock walls covered with vines. Our front lawn lay open to the street, which made our house somewhat modest, in an area where "modest" meant stately but slightly less than upper crust. My father had leveraged every asset we had to buy the house for $32,000 (it is probably worth more than $2 million U.S. now) because he wanted people to think our family was rich. We weren't.

To mark our early-winter move-in, he put up a twenty-five-foot Christmas tree. It climbed toward the peaked ceiling of the living room, which was the size of a basketball court. My three older sisters took turns clambering up a ladder to adorn the upper branches. My father shambled up the metal steps to place a star at the top. My younger sister and I, with our mother's coaching, sprinkled tinsel and placed ornaments on the bottom of the tree. There was peace in the family for a day.

Most days either my father was away working, playing bridge, or playing golf, or he was roaring at my mother and my three older sisters. He never drank alcohol, but he endured frequent migraine headaches. When a headache rolled in he would hunch over on a chair or couch. Then he would thunder around the house, hollering and smashing things. If I wasn't in his sight when the rages flared, I would scramble into any hiding place I could find and clamp my hands over my ears. Once my father broke my mother's hand, and she often wore bruises. He never hit me except for a lone spanking.

Sometimes he tried to play with me. After the peaceful day decorating the tree, I was thinking that maybe my father wasn't really a bad man. After all, he had suffered from polio as a child. He couldn't run around like me and had to spend his childhood in a hospital. And the morning after Christmas, when he tried out one of his presents, a new razor and set of blades, he proudly showed me the art of shaving. I watched in amazement as he stood before the mirror in the upstairs bathroom with his belly bulging over the top of his pajama bottoms. They covered his mangled left leg, which was sticklike from his childhood disease. While he was shaving, he cut his cheek, so he plastered it with a small bandage.

Later, when no one was looking, I tiptoed back up the stairs to the bathroom. I couldn't see myself in the mirror because I barely reached the top of the sink, but I ran the razor across my preschool cheeks. I scraped at the skin a few times and traipsed into the living room to show my family my handiwork. Blood poured down my face and spotted my blouse.

"What did you do?" my father shouted. He stormed and screamed and bellowed at me. I began to whimper and then to bawl. "Stop crying or I'll give you something to cry about," he roared. I pressed my lips together, trembling. He grabbed my arm and wrenched me up the winding staircase to the bathroom.

Snatching me around the waist, he lifted me up and forced my head into the sink under the running tap. Water washed through my hair and trickled pink over my face. I sputtered and sniveled and whined. "Stop crying!" he shouted again. I locked my mouth and willed my tears to stop.

Decades later, I wondered whether the razor cuts might have given me hepatitis C. The Centers for Disease Control and Prevention in the United States advises anyone with any kind of hepatitis not to share personal items that could carry their blood. These include razors. My father died in 2001, succumbing to heart disease, kidney failure, and cancer. I seldom talked with him about his illnesses, and I would never have thought to ask him whether his disease-riddled system was also harboring hep.

Often people infected with HCV (the hepatitis C virus) die from other causes, so there's a possibility he may have been infected. Because his childhood bout with polio had affected his leg, he underwent frequent surgery that required blood transfusions. Those surgeries would have occurred in the late 1920s or early '30s. Around that time transfusion blood was often collected from professional donors, who were told merely they should keep themselves in good physical condition, be careful about cleanliness, sleep in a well-ventilated room, and get daily exercise. They were never asked about hepatitis C. It wasn't even identified as a virus until 1989.

The U.S. Army reports that doctors in the '20s and '30s noticed "epidemic jaundice."[1] If some of that had been hepatitis C, my father may have had hep C most of his life. It may never have resulted in symptoms, since hepatology researchers report that the earlier in life you contract the virus, the longer it will take to seriously affect your liver. Although there is only a slim chance that I could have contracted the virus from my father's razor, it is possible. And if I had contracted it early in life, according to the research, that may be why I went for decades without symptoms.

## CHAPTER 2

# INTO THE FOG

THE SECOND TIME I visited Dr. Radev, the first thing I said to her was, "So I've got hemochromatosis?"

"No, it looks like something else," she said. "You need another test."

I was relieved that I might not to have to give blood frequently for the rest of my life, so I marched over to the lab without hesitation. I submitted another requisition to the medical assistant, lay on the cot, took a deep breath, clamped my eyes shut, and spread out my arm. The blood test was over in a literal pinch.

The idea that I might have "something else" sparked questions in my mind, but they fizzled away as I made plans for a vacation with Al in Mexico. Whatever the diagnosis was, it couldn't be too bad. I had always been healthy.

A week later I got another call from my doctor, asking me to come into the office. I thought she probably wanted to tell me about a minor problem the test had found, or maybe she just wanted to say I was 100 percent healthy.

The worst I expected to hear was that I had a vitamin deficiency or high cholesterol. Instead, Dr. Radev said, "You have antibodies to hepatitis C."

"What?"

"Hepatitis C," she said. "It's a disease that affects the liver."

I had heard about hepatitis C on the radio. I remembered listening to a documentary about a lawsuit over blood products that were infected with the virus, but other than that, I knew little about it.

"How could I have that?" I asked.

"You must have come into contact with it somehow. It's transmitted through blood," Dr. Radev said. Someone else's blood that carried the virus must have mixed with mine, she explained. She said that hep C could linger in the body for decades without showing symptoms. The virus might eventually scar the liver to the point that it would stop functioning. The result would be liver cancer or the need for a liver transplant.

"What?"

"Don't worry," she said in her soothing Philippine-accented voice. "About 20 percent of people who contract hepatitis C come down only with the acute form of the virus. It goes away on its own. People who just get acute hepatitis C may turn yellow or feel run-down for a few days or weeks, but their bodies fight off the infection. After that they no longer have the disease. They continue to produce antibodies for the rest of their life."

Dr. Radev asked if I had ever injected drugs. "No," I said.

She asked if I'd ever had surgery. "No," I said, "except for tonsils." She seemed puzzled (perhaps because tonsillectomies seldom require blood transfusions). She said that in rare instances hepatitis C can be transmitted through sex. I recalled that Jessica's father had once become jaundiced. Maybe Peter had contracted hepatitis C during his frequent flings and had passed the infection to me. "Jessica's father may have had hepatitis," I told Dr. Radev. "Maybe I got it from him."

But I had never become jaundiced, and I was a lot healthier than he had been. He got little exercise and was careless about his diet. I did lots of yoga and never ate junk food. Even if I had contracted the disease from him, I was sure I was among the 20 percent able to shake it off.

ACCORDING TO JULY 2016 figures from the World Health Organization, hepatitis C infects up to 150 million people worldwide and causes an estimated 700,000 deaths each year.[1] Between the United States and Canada, close to 3 million people are infected with hepatitis C. In 2015 Public Health England reported 214,000 cases in the UK, while Australia reported 230,500.

Despite these huge numbers, most people infected with hepatitis C don't know they have it. Many of them don't even remember they had any possible contact with the pathogen in their youth (the prime time to contract hep C) or suspect they might possibly carry the disease. I didn't, not even when my doctor said I had the antibodies.

Hepatitis has plagued humanity for thousands of years. The word *hepatitis* comes from a combination of the ancient Greek word *hepar,* meaning "liver," and the Latin word *itis,* meaning "inflammation." An epidemic of hepatitis was reported in China about five thousand years ago, and later an outbreak occurred in ancient Babylon. The Babylonians wrote of an illness that caused yellowing, fever, fatigue, and stomach problems. In Greece, in the first century BC,

Hippocrates referred to a disease that yellowed the skin. The Hippocratic Corpus, a library of ancient Greek medical writings by many authors, described hepatitis at least seven times and predicted the outcomes of the disease according to a person's degree of yellowness. In the second century AD, the Greek physician Aretaeus of Cappadocia studied the symptoms of hepatitis and wrote that the illness weakened "the liver's power of nutrition." Only recently has the yellowing disease been called *hepatitis* and been given alphabetical designations. In early 1969, when Peter's face turned yellow, the hepatitis alphabet had stalled at B. While I lay unconscious, waiting for a transfusion in 1971, the medical system had yet to screen donated blood for hepatitis C. Scientists didn't differentiate it from hep A or B until 1975.

Since that time, medical scientists have identified a string of viral diseases that attack the liver. The hepatitis alphabet now goes up to G. Each is a distinctive disease caused by a different pathogen:

- Hepatitis A: This is transmitted through food or water that is contaminated with feces. It's common in children. It is usually a mild disease and can be prevented by a vaccine.
- Hepatitis B: Like hepatitis C, it is transmitted through blood. It can also be spread through sex with an infected partner. Only 5 percent of cases become chronic. There is a vaccine for hepatitis B but no cure for the chronic illness.
- Hepatitis C: HCV is passed along through blood-to-blood contact. As Dr. Radev told me, about 20 percent of those who are infected experience only acute hepatitis C. These lucky people clear the infection with no treatment, but though they develop antibodies, they can

get reinfected. Another 80 percent of infected people develop the chronic form of the illness. Their infection continues until they die or are cured.

- Hepatitis D: This is a coinfection that occurs with hepatitis B. It causes severe liver disease.
- Hepatitis E: A common disease in India and many other developing countries, hepatitis E is transmitted through feces-contaminated food and water. It worsens any type of liver disease and may cause liver failure.
- Hepatitis F: This rare virus was found in 1994 in patients in Western Europe and India who had undergone blood transfusions. The virus was injected into rhesus monkeys and caused hepatitis. However, later studies suggested it was a mutation of the hepatitis B virus, and not all researchers recognize it as a distinct disease.
- Hepatitis G: This is transmitted through blood but isn't known to do harm to the *human* liver. The infection, which produces antibodies, is usually cleared within two years. One of the few studies on this virus showed that it can infect marmoset monkeys, which may suffer liver damage.

A healthy liver is mushy like a jellyfish. In reaction to the hepatitis virus, fibrosis ruffles through the liver, forming branches of scar tissue. In a healthy liver cell, DNA in the nucleus sends out RNA. The RNA tells the cell how to turn specific amino acids into healthy protein. But when the hep C virus invades the liver, it forces liver cells to make copies of itself instead. The virus reproduces incredibly fast, producing ten to the twelfth power (one million million) copies of itself each day.

The normal liver weighs just over two pounds and is the body's main blood-processing plant. It filters blood,

removing harmful substances, such as alcohol. It also manufactures proteins that defend against infection and help
the blood to clot; regulates the supply of vitamins, miner-
als, and hormones, including sex hormones; and produces,
stores, and regulates glucose and fat. It makes and elimi-
nates cholesterol and also converts it into lipoproteins that
deliver energy to the cells. Altogether, the liver performs
more than five hundred bodily functions. It continues to
do these jobs during the early stages of fibrosis, but later,
when the liver hardens into cirrhosis, it progressively loses
important abilities.

WHEN DR. RADEV told me I carried hep C antibodies, I
was so certain I had avoided the chronic form of the disease that even possible symptoms didn't worry me. I felt I
was healthy compared with friends who were aging in lock-
step with me. I believed my joint problems came from a
car accident many years before. I believed my acid reflux
came from doing too much yoga, which I thought had
pulled my esophagus out of place. I thought my muddy
mind came from lack of sleep caused by the joint pain and
from overwork, which retirement would cure. These were
all mechanical lifestyle problems. A nasty virus could never
get me, I believed.

Dr. Radev said an acute case of hepatitis C might seem
like the flu. I recalled that about a year after I had noted
Peter's yellowness, we both came down with an awful flu.

Was it really the flu? Maybe it was hep, I thought as I
left Dr. Radev's office. Peter and I had both probably experienced the acute form of hep, I reasoned, and our flu-like
symptoms were its manifestation. Now I was safe from
the hep C virus forever. In fact, I was so confident I was
healthy that the next week I submitted a formal letter to

my employer. I'd be resigning from work as a teacher—and from a gold-plated medical plan that most people with hepatitis C would envy. I planned to celebrate my coming retirement with a vacation.

It was the end of the spring 2014 semester. I had been having trouble with my jobs, one at a university and the other at a college, so I had taken a partial leave. Together, the jobs involved teaching four courses to a total of ninety-plus students. I had been finding it hard to switch my mind from one topic to the next and from one student to the next. That had been easy in the past, but now it seemed inordinately complex and stressful. I was experiencing severe arm and shoulder pain at night. I thought the pain caused my sleeplessness, which in turn impaired my ability to multitask. The problem went beyond teaching and into my home life. The last couple of years before I knew I had hep C, I had begun to feel edgy any time I had to tackle more than one activity at a time. When my cell phone chimed while I was paying bills online, tremors would climb into my shoulders. One day I was putting socks on my dog, Zeena, to protect her chronic sore feet, and my husband asked about ferry times. Thinking about two tasks together made me jumpy. I scowled at Zeena and tried to hide my irritation from Al. Zeena loved the comfort of socks, but she must have sensed that something was wrong. She struggled to get away from me, twisting and yelping. Al glanced over and said, "Go easy on her." Later I was sorting laundry and he asked for the car keys. I shouted, "Not now!" Similar scenes occurred again and again.

The most irritating task was cooking. Chefs, homemakers, and occasional cooks should know that preparing a balanced, several-course meal and serving everything on time, warm but not charred, can be one of the most complex multitasking exercises in the universe. I had always enjoyed cooking healthful, many-course meals. But with hepatitis C swimming though my system, inflaming my organs, and sending crazy messages to my glands, something went awry. One day a couple of friends came by and I volunteered to make dinner. I decided to prepare chicken with mushroom sauce, broccoli, and a salad. I had to time the chicken in the oven, stir and watch the sauce, cut and steam the broccoli, slice and dice veggies for salad, press a couple of garlic cloves, mix an oil and vinegar salad dressing, and toss the salad. Making sure each dish appeared at the same time on the table was too much for me. I grumbled at Al as he watched me chopping tomatoes at the cutting board. Our friends were outside on the deck, and I was glad they couldn't see me as I bashed my elbow into the salad dressing, which splattered all over the counter.

In the meantime, the sauce for the chicken was burning. I lunged at the stove to turn down the heat and barked at Al, waking a snoozing Zeena, who looked at me as if I were a strange, threatening animal. Al wisely left the kitchen. As I checked the sauce again, I burned my palm and spilled half of the lumpy liquid on the floor. The guests were now chatting twenty feet away in the living room. Fortunately, they didn't notice the gooey spoon I hurled at the floor and my muffled cry of "Crap!"

While I could hide most of my edginess at home, I had a hard time concealing it from students. One of the joys of teaching had been getting to know them personally. I had discovered early in my career that once I knew a bit about individual students, I would like them, which would motivate me toward better teaching. During the first class, I would ask students about their hobbies, part-time jobs, travels, and ambitions. As they took turns introducing themselves, I would memorize their names and distinctive qualities.

In the past I had learned two-thirds of my students' names as they chatted on that first day of class, and I'd learn the other third within a week or two. But during the two years before my diagnosis, it seemed there were far too many names to learn at once. I become increasingly unable to remember who was Jean and who was James. I couldn't recall which student bred labradoodles, which one worked as a house painter, and which in which class came from Thailand. By the middle of the semester, the year before I learned I had hep, I could recall only five or six names out of the ninety-four students I taught. It was maddening.

The semester before my diagnosis, I decided to give up on the memory work. Why try to remember names when you know you'll forget them in an instant? It got to the point that when a student raised a hand, I'd just nod. It wasn't a great way to establish rapport. I started drawing little pictures of my students' faces on index cards. I added arrows to facial features and labeled them "honey-brown hair" or "squinty eyes" and made notes such as "born Thailand, high school England, trekked through Italy with her dad." That helped somewhat, but it was hard to riffle through a stack of cards when a student or two raised their hands.

I knew I didn't have Alzheimer's because my grandmother, who was stricken with the illness, experienced different memory problems. Her memory lapses had been like sudden gaping holes that filled themselves with confusion and hurled her backward into earlier times. I remember visiting my parents' home in Manhasset, a chichi suburb of New York City. I had just reconnected with my parents after avoiding them for almost a decade. My grandmother, in her late seventies, had moved in with them so they could help her through her dementia. In her lucid moments she was a jolly white-haired lady, but those moments could dissipate fast. Once she took me to her room and pulled a shoe box from under her bed. "I've got some nice ribbons for you. You can wear them in your hair," she said, yanking a tangle of ribbons from the box.

"Thank you," I said, unraveling a length of inch-wide blue satin. "This one's nice."

She grabbed it from me. The kindness in her face evaporated and fury replaced it. "You've been stealing from me! Give that back," she wailed. Later that day she dressed in her finest blouse, hat, and gloves, and she slipped out the door. My mother found her wandering along a sidewalk a few blocks away in a neighborhood of sprawling single-family homes, muttering, "I'm looking to rent an apartment. Where is the apartment building?"

No, I didn't have Alzheimer's. I was just getting to be an absent-minded professor, I decided. But I didn't like the situation, so I would move on. I started planning my retirement from teaching. Later, after hearing I had hep, I realized my teaching problems had come from brain fog, a common complaint of people with hepatitis C—and one that usually vanishes after treatment.

IN SPRING 2014, I wanted to get far away from work so that I could put my head back together, so to speak. Flights to Cancun were cheap from Vancouver, and the eastern strip of the Yucatán Peninsula seemed to be just the place to go for R&R. I still thought my cloudy thinking came solely from pain-caused sleep deprivation. I had been getting less than three hours' sleep a night, not enough to enter deep, slow-wave sleep, without which the memory suffers. I imagined that having nothing to do under a hot Mexican sun would lull me into prolonged slumber. I would enjoy a mindless vacation and regain my mind. I knew nothing yet about brain fog and little about hepatitis C, and I was certain that other than having an unrelenting case of fatigue, I was as healthy as a puppy. So I booked the flights and a stay at a resort near Akumal, Mexico.

The resort curled through lush, tropical forest along a white-sand lagoon on the Yucatán Peninsula about halfway between Playa del Carmen and the Mayan ruins at Tulum, with swimming pools, pyramid-shaped residences, restaurants, tiki bars, poolside bars, and beach bars. Part of the relaxation I sought was the sleep inducement of free-flowing liquor, which was included in the resort fee.

We arrived around midnight at the Cancun Airport. The cab that picked us up drove sluggishly along the Mayan Riviera highway and crawled slower than a snail through a Federales roadblock along the route. Finally, the cab turned into the resort's winding entry road, which was shrouded with palm trees lit from below by spotlights. We shuffled up the grand staircase and past a wall of blue glass into the lobby. The desk clerk said we had missed the dinner buffet, so we strolled into a bar in the main building. A band played contemporary rock. About a hundred people milled about. A few were dancing, but most were drinking. The bar reached along one of the walls, where eight bartenders poured every color of alcohol, ceaselessly. I slid onto a stool and asked for a drink. It was the first of quarts of margaritas I downed at the resort. For someone like me who tends to avoid in-pool volleyball games and goofy poolside contests designed for kids, there wasn't much to do. So I did what most visitors did most of the time at the resort: eat, swim, and drink. I must have drunk at least forty alcoholic beverages during our five-day visit.

When we arrived back home, I left my bags scattered on the living-room floor and walked out onto the deck that runs the length of our home. The phone rang, but I didn't bother to go inside to pick it up.

Four days later I dialed my voice mail, and a message asked me to call Dr. Radev's office. After a blurry week on the Riviera Maya, the threat of having hep antibodies had slipped my mind. I figured that since Dr. Radev was new as my doctor, her office probably wanted information about me they had yet to collect. I waited another few days before I called back. Exactly one week after the end of my vacation, I poured a morning mug of coffee and dialed the doctor's number. "You called last week?" I asked.

"Doctor Radev wants you to come in," a pleasant voice said.

"How about two weeks from today?"

"We can take you much sooner," the medical receptionist said.

"When?"

"Today?"

"No. I can't make it." I sipped some coffee.

"Could you be here Friday morning or early afternoon?"

"How about Monday?"

"There's an opening first thing in the morning. How about 8:45?"

"Sure," I said. I was pleased that Dr. Radev's schedule had so many open times, when I was used to having to book two weeks ahead for a doctor's appointment. The spacious waiting room had been buzzing with patients the last time I was there. A lot of her patients must already have left for summer vacations, I thought.

I was wrong. I learned that Dr. Radev wanted me to come in as soon as possible because my situation was pressing. At 8:45 a.m. Monday, May 12, I sat in her examining room. Dr. Radev took a long breath, lowered her voice, and said, "You have hepatitis C."

# GROUPIE

DURING THE DECADES between the razor cuts and my father's death, I avoided not only bloodletting but my father as well. In high school my strategy for this was to become a groupie. The pastime required a lengthy bus and subway trip that kept me away from home the maximum amount of time my parents would allow. On most days after school I would travel from Queens into Manhattan with a few other girls. We would gather in front of a midtown hotel and wait for Herman's Hermits or the Moody Blues to show up. Then we would try to sneak into the hotel. A pack of doormen usually kept us out.

One night, returning from a round of rock-star stalking, three friends and I jumped onto a subway car. The theaters had just got out, so it was hard to find a seat. My friends reached for straps that hung from the ceiling. I was too short to grasp the swaying loops, so I edged through clumps of passengers to the floor-to-ceiling pole between the exit doors. A tall young blond guy clung to the same pole as me. As the train chugged and lurched, my head bumped his shoulder. He looked like Richard Chamberlain, my favorite actor, who starred in the TV series *Dr. Kildare*. We started talking. Kevin told me he was a musician. When the train stopped at his station in Jackson Heights, I raced out the door with him. My groupie friends looked on, dismayed. Kevin gave me a tour of his neighborhood that night, and within a few weeks we were going steady.

Because I had skipped third grade, I graduated from high school at age sixteen. I found a job as a file clerk for the head office of the Allegheny Ludlum Steel Company on Park Avenue.

I was soon promoted to switchboard operator and then teletype operator. After work, sometimes I'd meet my friends in the East Village, where hippies would give us flowers or offer us a joint. While roaming through the area one day, I saw a For Rent sign on the window of a ground-level apartment. I rang the superintendent's bell, and a scraggly-haired woman in coveralls stumbled out. When I asked her if I could rent the place, she gazed at my work attire and nodded. I exchanged that week's pay envelope for a set of keys.

Back in Flushing, confronting my parents in the living room, I said, "I've got my own apartment. I need the thousand dollars you owe me." They had held the money in trust from a settlement I had received after having been thrown to the floor in a car accident as a child.

"What? Not on your life," my father said, making squishing sounds on the plastic-covered sofa where he sat.

"You're too young to be on your own," my mother said, also making squishing sounds.

"You told me you wanted me to leave when I graduated. I'm doing exactly what you asked."

"You're not getting the money," my father said. He limped around the coffee table, scowling at me.

"It's my money." I backed away from him.

"Not on your life, you little slut," my father said.

That inspired me. I said, "I need money to buy furniture. I guess I'll have to stand on a street corner and earn it the way the sluts do."

My parents gave me the money. In mid-October 1966, two weeks after my seventeenth birthday, I moved into the bachelor suite on East 6th Street. I decorated it with a thousand dollars' worth of furniture. In those days a thousand dollars went far. I bought a table, chairs, dressers, and a convertible sofa to sleep on, and I splurged on a spiffy, curved-front TV, a hi-fi, and even a reel-to-reel tape recorder. I hung hand-printed Indian tapestries on the walls. Kevin came by to help me get organized. Being a newly independent hormone-filled teen, I invited him to spend the night. We fumbled at our early attempts at sex, but my hormones were happy and Kevin didn't want to leave. I said I had planned to live alone, but he objected. I had been morphing from a miniskirted groupie into a Village-style hippie who wore waist-length hair and tie-dyed shirts. After a few more fumblings with Kevin, I figured I might as well do as the hippies did. Cohabitation was becoming the norm. "I guess we're living together," I said, but that didn't mean we'd have a sexual free-for-all.

Kevin grew up in a Roman Catholic family. He spent time as an altar boy and often listened to priests who railed that sex was for procreation only. He was eighteen when he moved in with me, and the missionary position was his only position.

My parents cooled down and I visited them for Christmas. In January they came to see my apartment. Kevin answered the door. My mother's face paled and my father's grew stern. They left without speaking to me. To my surprise, within weeks they were planning a wedding. Kevin and I were relieved. A priest in my Catholic high school had recommended the rhythm method of birth control. Kevin and I had practiced it, but it didn't work. I had always wanted to be a mom, so I was happy.

Kevin—at first—fulfilled my parents' key requirement for a husband: he had an income. His band, the Inner Sanctum, was appearing in the musical *The Golden Screw* at the Provincetown Playhouse in Greenwich Village and getting union rates as actors. We got married within a month at the famed celebrity hangout Sardi's and had a write-up in *Variety*. Around that time, I hit the iron ceiling at the steel company. Only men could be promoted to the sales desk. Thinking *The Golden Screw* was truly golden, I quit my job. But the off-Broadway musical closed a week after the wedding. Kevin was now an unemployed rock musician with a pregnant wife. We could barely afford the $87 a month rent on our East Village bachelor suite or the $15 a week it took to buy groceries. Kevin said he would sell his blood and contended that I should become a paid donor too.

"I can't do that," I said, patting my soon-to-grow tummy. I was seventeen and pregnant. I was relieved to have an excuse.

IN THE 1960s in New York City, people who sold a pint of their blood would receive between $5 and $200, depending on blood type. Kevin discovered he could get $50. Soon, though, he found a job as a shipping clerk with *Sun and Health* magazine. He spent his work days wrapping and mailing magazines. He brought stacks of them home, where we gawked together at photos of nudists playing volleyball and basking on the sand, wearing nothing but sun hats and sandals. Kevin also began bringing home a paycheck and didn't have to get his blood siphoned for money.

It might have been good if he had, though. As far as I know he didn't have hepatitis, and his blood might have saved someone from getting it. Dr. Harvey Alter, from the National Institutes of Health in the United States, explained in a BioCentury TV webcast in 2014 that in those days people who received blood from volunteers rather than paid donors had only a 7 percent chance of contracting hepatitis. Even a 7 percent chance of getting hep would be scary, but it was a lot better at the time than the 30 percent rate for all blood transfusions.

While Kevin worked at *Sun and Health,* I found a job as a page at MGM Records, where I traipsed from room to room delivering documents. I remember watching Petula Clark stroll down a hallway and seeing Frank Zappa and other kooky rock stars cavort in the employee cafeteria. I loved the job, but in those days, women could be fired for being pregnant. It was the time of loose-fitting sack dresses, so I took to wearing extreme examples of the fashion. Nonetheless, co-workers began to stare at me.

I told Kevin I'd have to quit my job. His job hardly paid our rent, and he again suggested he'd donate blood. Just in time, his agent got the Inner Sanctum a gig opening for the Velvet Underground. Once again there would be no blood selling.

A lot of other people were selling their blood, however. There were countless thousands of paid donors in the sixties, many of them prisoners and those who needed cash to support drug habits. Their blood would kill many future transfusion recipients, whose livers would fail because the donors' blood carried hepatitis C.

I gave birth to Della two days before my eighteenth birthday. Six weeks later, my doctor suggested I go on birth control pills. That was the first time I had heard about them. I went to the Planned Parenthood clinic and fainted while the nurse was drawing blood.

## CHAPTER 3

# TAINTED TOOLS

D R. RADEV'S VOICE sounded fuzzy. I stared at the vinyl surface of the examining table. I felt as if I had been swept into the Phantom Zone—the alternate dimension in Superman comics where outlaws from Krypton are banished and serve their sentences as insubstantial beings. They can observe our universe but are invisible to anyone in it. Drawings of the Phantom Zone often depict its inmates howling for mercy with their eyes bulging in fear. As the diagnosis shrouded my consciousness, I must have looked like the most tortured criminal from Krypton.

"What?" I asked. "I thought I only had antibodies."

Dr. Radev said when someone contracts hepatitis C, the immune system produces antibodies that specifically attack the virus. The blood continues to make them, regardless of whether the person kicks the disease. "I'll send you to an excellent specialist," she said. "He does clinical trials, and he knows all about the latest treatments. There are some new, very effective drugs being developed."

"Oh, good," I mumbled.

"The new treatments can be very expensive," she said.

"Expensive" made me think the drugs might cost $10,000. I soon learned that the newest treatment cost well over $100,000—one thousand percent of my guesstimate (that was in 2014). That would kill my travel budget for fifteen years. I was sure my extended medical plan covered prescription drugs, but I would soon be leaving my job and the plan. It was too late to take back my resignation. I'd have to move quickly toward whatever treatment I needed. "When can I see the specialist?" was my number one question.

Dr. Radev said she would send him a note explaining that I needed quick treatment. If my insurance wouldn't cover it, she said, I might be able to get into a clinical trial.

I had recently read the novel *The Normals* by David Gilbert. In it, an unemployed recent Harvard grad signs up for a paid drug trial. He lives for many weeks at a drug-company campus. The book describes a prison-like setting with oddball participants, uncaring nurses, and appalling side effects. The plot was meant to be funny, but it scared the bejesus out of me. Why would I want to get into a clinical trial? I could wind up with a placebo, I thought, and never get rid of my disease. I'd later learn that placebos were seldom involved in hep C drug studies. Instead, the trials tend to compare different treatments in terms of cure rates and side effects. But in Dr. Radev's office the suggestion of a clinical trial made me squirm. I didn't even think of asking the specialist's name.

"He will need to know your genotype first," Dr. Radev said.

The genotype test is a blood test. I winced at the thought of it, but I was afraid to waste a second while the virus was building demon roads through my liver. I raced out of the clinic and ran across the parking lot to the lab.

In the two weeks between the time I heard I had hep and the time I learned my genotype, I talked with my closest family about my illness. My husband, my two daughters, and my two sons-in-law were ultra-nice and ultra-concerned. My grandchildren, a preteen girl and a teenage boy, heard about the hep as they listened to family conversations, and they were ultra-nice too. Everyone got tested for hepatitis C. Despite family habits that included occasional toothbrush sharing with my husband, I was the only one infected.

Sharing household items that come in contact with hep-tainted blood is on the list of possible means of transmission. In a study published in 2006, a team of eight researchers from the University of Regensburg in Germany found that twelve out of thirty patients who had hep showed small amounts of HCV-RNA in their toothbrush-rinsing water. The study concluded that there is a "theoretical risk of infection by sharing these objects."[1] Another study, from Spain, published in the journal *Oral Diseases*, noted that specific receptors for the virus have not been found in the mouth and HCV particles in saliva are not very infectious. The German team summed it up:

> The mere finding of HCV-RNA on the surface of contaminated tools does not prove potential transmission of the virus by these tools, of course, and the low infection risk usually published for household contacts of hepatitis C patients provides good evidence against a significant role of transmission by household objects.[2]

Still, when I was diagnosed, I did what I could to discourage borrowing. I get lots of guests in the summer. One of them might have a toothbrush that looks like mine. I moved my toothbrush to a cabinet where a guest couldn't find it and left new, packaged toothbrushes on the bathroom counter for anyone to use.

When I talked with other people who had hep, I learned they took a similar approach. John Lavette, a retired flower merchant, came down with hep C while living the hippie life in Haight-Ashbury. Hippies tended to share everything, but when John learned he had hepatitis C, he became strictly personal with his toiletries. "When someone asks to borrow my toothbrush, I tell people, 'Use your finger, dude. You're not putting my toothbrush in your mouth,'" he said. "A friend recently asked me, 'When you shave with a razor, something like a Bic, do you throw it out?' I said, 'I've thrown them out for the last ten years.'"

Andrew Loog Oldham, manager of the Rolling Stones from 1963 to 1967, is also scrupulous about not sharing anything that has even a tiny chance of picking up blood. His list of items is longer than John's and includes cocaine straws. In the sixties, lines of cocaine were often laid out on tables at rock stars' parties for guests like Andrew to snort.

He and I sat across from each other drinking chai on the patio of Terra Breads In Vancouver's Olympic Village. Andrew had just come back from Pilates and Rolfing and was wearing a black T-shirt with a gold herringbone pattern across the front. Wispy white hair accentuated the narrowness of his face. His hazel eyes were framed by pouches on the bottom and thin eyebrows that arched so close to his eyes, I couldn't see the lids. His shoulders were square and erect. He appeared to be in great physical shape for a seventy-year-old man, especially one with hepatitis C.

He must have been cool and handsome when he managed the rhythm and blues band, I mused. I thought back to a summer day when I was fourteen, when I milled among a crowd of sixty groupies in front of the Hotel Century on

47th Street near Times Square. The Rolling Stones' limousine rolled out of a parking garage and stopped, waiting to make a turn. A horde of screaming teenagers rushed the car. They pressed against its shaded windows, trying to glimpse their idols. I lurched closest to the back of the limo. The other girls pushed forward. They bashed me into the bumper and pushed me atop the trunk. More than ten other girls piled on top of me, smacking my face against the rear window of the car. Brian Jones sat in the back seat. He scowled at me. He rapped his fist against the inside of the window right at my face. He pummeled the window again and again. His silky blond hair swayed as he pounded at me through the glass. The window vibrated. The car began to move. Gradually it moved faster. Gradually the other girls fell away. Last, I slipped off the back of the car. I was shaking and breathing hard. I had thought I might be run over, but only my knees were bruised from hitting the pavement.

I thought Andrew would have been in the limo with the Stones that day and couldn't have missed the incident. I asked him whether he had seen me getting bumped about against the window.

"Well, I don't know," Andrew said. He had traveled the world with the Stones and had encountered countless mobs of groupies. He was partying a lot in those days, he said, and many scenes had become a blur to him.

In the heyday of rock 'n' roll he hobnobbed not only with the Rolling Stones but also with many other rock stars whose music he had promoted or produced. His label, Immediate Records, produced music by Eric Clapton, John Mayall, Small Faces, Fleetwood Mac, Rod Stewart, and Nico, whom I had hung out with at the Scene nightclub in New York when my first husband's band opened for hers (and Lou Reed's), the Velvet Underground. I'd had a taste of the rock 'n' roll party life, but Andrew Loog Oldham had consumed the full meal, imbibing, snorting, and injecting all sorts of drugs, including heroin and cocaine.

Eventually Andrew decided to get healthy and visited an alternative health care practitioner in Glens Falls, New York, who was associated with Scientology. Andrew and his wife, Esther, began taking Scientology courses, and Andrew asked to sign up for a Purification Rundown. The process, according to its designer, Scientology founder L. Ron Hubbard, would purge the body of toxins, including those from IV drug use and LSD. Andrew was refused the treatment because he had once received shock therapy, so he visited another alternative medical man, who prescribed a similar toxin-cleansing regimen. For a month or two Andrew ingested huge amounts of niacin (vitamin B3). "You start off on 50 or 100 milligrams of niacin, and by the time you're finished you're up to 5,000 milligrams a day— and that is not good for a compromised liver," he said as he pushed down the plunger on a Bodum of tea. In fact, high doses of niacin have been linked to severe and even fatal liver injury.

About two years later Andrew returned to the practitioner, who tested his muscles. Andrew, reading upside down, saw "hep C?" on the doctor's note sheet. He asked the doctor why he had written that.

"He said, 'I'm wondering if you have hep C,'" Andrew recalled. "I said, 'Well, I'll go and get tested.' So I did."

In 1997 he learned he did have hepatitis C. Testing revealed 4 million bits of HCV in each milliliter of his blood. He visited more than one doctor who suggested treatment with interferon. "I never went back because I didn't trust them," Andrew said.

He said he knows a famous Spanish singer who tried to cure his hep C with interferon, and after five months the man's marriage nearly broke up from the stress of treatment. Another friend told him, "Don't you dare. My mother died from interferon." On top of knowing about the horrible side effects of the drug, Andrew learned he was infected with hepatitis genotype 1a. Unlike some other types of hep C, which could be treated back then for twenty-four weeks, Andrew would have to do interferon for a year. "Instinctively, I didn't want to go near it," he said.

He carried on with alternative medicine. Sometimes he would go to four practitioners at a time. "I've been as obsessive about wellness as I was about unwellness," he told me. He said alternative medicine helped him for at least eighteen years after he contracted hep, which he believed occurred in the 1980s.

Of many possible ways he may have acquired hep C, Andrew said, he suspects a tube he used to snort cocaine was the culprit. He said Tiffany's jewelers used to sell cocaine straws for $175, which was a lot of money for most people in the eighties but not much for Andrew's high-rolling friends. Andrew described the party toy as a shiny tube of silver, eight to ten inches long. Because it was so long, it often clogged up. He and his friends would scrape out the cocaine with paper clips. The straw could have had anybody's blood on it, which may have given him hepatitis, Andrew said.

While blood could conceivably get on a razor or on a cocaine straw and transmit hepatitis C, transmission through medical tools is far more common. In fact, medical tools were the most common method of transmission until the mid-1990s. Historically, worldwide, most hepatitis C infections have been passed along by inadvertent medical exposure. Someone who has hep gets treated at an underequipped medical unit or mobile clinic; syringes, tubes, or vessels don't get sterilized properly; and zing— that person's hep C seeps into another person's blood. It can be passed along through the same or other routes ad infinitum . . . or until everyone in the branching trail has been cured.

THE FIRST REPORTED incidence of the spread of hepatitis though contaminated medical tools occurred in 1883 in Bremen, Germany, at a shipbuilding company. A public health inspector discovered that hepatitis had been spread through cowpox inoculations that took place at the factory. Doctors collected and mixed the discharge from many patients who had cowpox, a mild disease, and the fluid was applied to scrapes on people's skin to protect them against smallpox. About two hundred workers at the shipbuilding factory came down with hepatitis, out of thirteen hundred who had been inoculated.

During World War II, at least 26,771 soldiers who received a vaccine for yellow fever came down with hepatitis. It was hard to sterilize syringes, especially on the battlefield, where conditions were brutal and unpredictable. Close to 200,000 cases of hepatitis were reported among U.S. soldiers. Not long after the war—in 1950—transmission of the disease reached its peak.

The first disposable syringes, introduced in the 1950s, should have prevented most transmission of the disease in medical settings, but sloppy medical practices still occurred sporadically, especially in underdeveloped countries. In 2010 a study in Brazil of 256 blood donors showed a high probability that dental patients would acquire hepatitis C from improperly sterilized instruments. Aside from the home use of syringes among the patients, root canals and surgical removal of tartar were cited as the main methods of transmission.

From the 1950s to the 1980s, Egypt carried out a program to vaccinate people against schistosomiasis, also known as bilharzia and commonly called "snail fever." The disease is spread by parasitic flatworms that live in freshwater snails that burrow into the skin of swimmers. The flatworms enter the person's blood vessels and lay eggs that can attach to body tissues, usually in veins that drain the intestines or the urinary tract. About 240 million people worldwide suffer from snail fever. Each year more than 200,000 people die from the disease. Egypt's vaccination campaign used contaminated needles and syringes, and hepatitis C spread throughout the populace. As a result, at least 10 percent of Egyptians aged fifteen to fifty-nine became infected with hepatitis C.[3]

Vietnam is also high on the World Health Organization's hepatitis C crisis list because of faulty medical practices. Jenny Heathcote, winner of the 2015 University Health Network Global Impact Award for her work in hepatology, told medical students that in Vietnam "there are so many outbreaks, the health system doesn't bother screening for the virus."[4]

Western nations have spread the virus through contaminated medical equipment too. The Centers for Disease Control and Prevention in the United States reported that between 2008 and 2015, ninety-six patients were infected with hepatitis C at hemodialysis clinics in eighteen separate outbreaks. In Canada, Dr. Gary Garber, chief of infection prevention and control for Public Health Ontario, told me he had noticed a disturbing trend. In several colonoscopy clinics, patients had contracted hepatitis C. When a new case of hep C arises in someone who has no risk factors, the agency goes through the patient's medical history. "An investigator probably said, 'Oh isn't that interesting? The person had a colonoscopy. Two patients before them had hepatitis C,'" Garber said to me on the phone.[5]

In a specific 2014 case, Waterloo Region Public Health investigated a case of hep C in a patient who had no risk factors other than a visit to a colonoscopy clinic the day before Christmas. The agency then found another patient with hep C who went through the same procedure on the same day at the same clinic. The investigation turned up another three infected patients who had visited the Tri-City Colonoscopy Clinic on Christmas Eve. The genetic makeup of the virus in all five cases was too similar to be a coincidence. Eight other patients treated that day were virus free. So were the clinic's staff members. No specific means of transmission was found in the clinic. The health agency worked with the clinic to improve its techniques, and the clinic stayed open.[6]

This was a relatively small medical outbreak compared with one that happened in Nebraska. In 2000 and 2001, ninety-nine cancer patients at a chemotherapy clinic at the Fremont Area Medical Center came down with an odd strain of hepatitis C. The oncologist who had treated them blamed the outbreak on patients' previous behaviors. But all of the patients tested with the same genotype, 3a, a rare genotype in the United States, suggesting a common means of transmission. Investigators discovered that a nurse in the clinic had reused bags of saline (apparently, to save money). Hep-tainted blood passed from patient to patient through the saline used to flush their chemotherapy ports. Dr. Tahir Javed, who ran the clinic, knew of the practices yet allowed them to go on. During the investigation,

Javed fled to his native country, Pakistan, where he was subsequently appointed health minister. Later he surrendered his medical license for Nebraska.

According to Evelyn V. McKnight, one of the ninety-nine patients, there was a cover-up. The hospital—where McKnight's husband practiced medicine—tried to quash any mention of the hep-tainted medical bags, but ultimately the courts sided with McKnight. In 2014 she and lawyer Travis T. Bennington coauthored *The Never Event,* which reported that sixteen of the ninety-nine patients— about one in six—progressed to advanced liver disease.

Those odds scared me. Granted, the unfortunate sixteen in Nebraska had suffered from compromised immune systems because of their cancer therapy. But McKnight compiled her statistics after less than fifteen years. The long-term odds of cirrhosis for anyone with hepatitis C are worse. Of the 80 percent of infected people who develop the chronic form of the illness, 20 percent develop cirrhosis after twenty years. By thirty years it's 41 percent. After that, according to renowned hep C researcher Jordan Feld, it's likely to go up to 50 to 60 percent. Each year, 1 to 4 percent of people with cirrhosis are diagnosed with liver cancer. That was my big fear. Was I on the way to a cure or something else? I didn't yet know.

1968–1969

# HIPPIE

IN THE FALL of 1968, I hooked up with Peter, who had attended
the same high school as I had. He had been popular at Bayside
High, while I, except for my camaraderie with groupie friends—
mostly from other schools—had been a quiet, studious girl who
kept to herself. I would sit in the park across the street from
school and pretend to read a book, sneaking looks at the cool
kids who lounged against the chain-link fence that surrounded
the basketball court. Peter always seemed to be the center of
attention. I noticed his broad shoulders, his thick black hair
(which began to recede a few years later), and the confident grin
on his face. He had thin eyebrows for a boy and a bronze, wide-
cheeked face he had inherited from his Indigenous grandmother.
He was brawny but not what I'd call cute—my key requirement
for boyfriends back then. In fact, were it not for Peter's bravado
and popularity, I never would have hooked up with him a few
years later. And I probably would not have acquired hepatitis. But
I wouldn't have had my daughter Jessica, which would have been
a giant shame.

During the two years after I graduated, I married a rock musician, had a baby, held several office jobs, painted murals, and
lived in Woodstock for a summer, performing in a comedy Western theater troupe. Peter had married a woman and left her with
a daughter who had been born with cerebral palsy. He joined the
army. After basic training he heard he'd be going to Vietnam, so
he deserted.

Around the time he left the army, I left my husband. Kevin
had quit his job at the nudist magazine and chosen to stay home

in our East Village railroad flat, playing guitar while I worked at an office job. I had to leave Della with a babysitter because he refused to change diapers. When I arrived home each day, Kevin expected me to do all of the housework—or else he would whine or start a fight. He insisted that I darn his socks like his mother had. He would stare at a blank wall for an hour each day, chanting *om mani padme hūm*. I asked him why he was chanting.

"I need a new guitar," he said as he backed away from the wall. "If I chant, the universe will give me a Stratocaster." I reasoned I had signed up for one child but not for two, so one day while Kevin was out practicing with his band, I left a good-bye note, scooped up my daughter, and took the Long Island Rail Road to my parents' home in Queens.

Within days I met—or re-met—Peter. I was talking with my friend Diane at a little triangular park near the tracks when Peter arrived with some hippie men. He said hi to Diane, and she introduced us. Peter didn't remember me from high school. I didn't mention my fantasies about him. He asked where I lived, and I strategically said, "The East Village," which was considered very cool. He motioned toward one of the playground swings. "Give it a try," he said. I hopped onto the child-height seat and raised my legs to avoid the ground. Peter pushed me. I knew right off that he liked me. I flew high, secretly proud of the attention I was getting from the popular boy of my high school years.

Soon Peter and I moved in together, and soon after that we left New York City to live in the U.S. Virgin Islands. We believed the islands were so remote that the army would never find him.

The Virgin Islands are part of the Lesser Antilles archipelago, which comprises many islands and island clusters. Some are sovereign nations and others are governed separately under the dominions of France, the UK, the Netherlands, Venezuela, and the United States. We chose the U.S. territory because we wouldn't need passports to enter. Peter, our friends Ryan and

Harry, toddler Della, and I flew into idyllic St. Thomas just after New Year's in 1969. We rented a one-bedroom suite for all five of us and slept on air mattresses on the floor. At first I got a job as a secretary. Then I realized Peter's and Ryan's night-time jobs at restaurants let them spend their days at the beach, so I became a server at the Pirate's Pub. It was the hangout for American sailors who hadn't seen a woman in months. I would come home at three in the morning with black and blue spots all over my backside from where they had pinched me.

But the bruises were worth it. I hung out at Coki Point Beach every day. I spooned sand into plastic buckets with Della, snorkeled through sapphire-clear water chasing angelfish, and wrote letters to hippie friends about the bliss of the islands. Many of them flew down from New York. We rented a second apartment. We shared our paychecks with the new arrivals, who lazed on the beach every day and never found jobs. Ryan, Peter, and I supported seven adult hippies and two babies. When our cash ran short, Peter took on longer shifts at the restaurant, but that didn't help much.

One day I called my parents from a phone booth.

"Come home and we'll buy you a restaurant," my father said.

"We could make money in New York, come back here, and buy some land," I posited to Peter.

"But the army?"

"We'll own the restaurant. You can be off the books."

That sealed it. We would head back to New York City. I was sure we'd make enough money in a year or two to return to the islands and buy our own paradise cottage on a beach.

Soon after we returned to New York, I noticed Peter's island tan was fading into a yellow tint. His face appeared particularly sallow. He complained of a stomach upset and odd, light-colored stools, which are signs of liver disease. I didn't know it then, but Peter may have contracted hepatitis.

In our cramped little island home, we had all had just a hot plate and sink, and we didn't keep much to eat there other than bread, eggs, tinned milk, and sardines. That was about all the few stores on St. Thomas regularly carried. Peter often ate at the busy hotel where he worked. Food was free for staff, and many different co-workers prepared the meals. Health inspections in the Virgin Islands at the time may have been less scrupulous than those in the mainland U.S., so hepatitis could have traveled through the kitchen staff.

When I was diagnosed, I did not yet know the difference between hep A and hep C, and I figured Peter must have picked up hepatitis C from food handling. Was it possible that the demon could have entered my blood through him?

## CHAPTER 4

# FLUS AND ACCIDENTS

SOON AFTER MY diagnosis, I learned Peter's jaundice was probably from hepatitis A rather than C. The A disease has similar symptoms to other types of hepatitis, but it usually leaves the body no worse than it was before. Hepatitis A is generally passed through contact with feces. That happens more than you may think. Often preschool children, who have yet to learn the niceties of toilet training, contract and pass along hepatitis A at daycare centers. Their parents might never know their kids were sick. People can also contract hep A from poor bathroom hygiene combined with food handling. One person preparing food can transmit the disease to hundreds of others. The good news is that hepatitis A generally lasts only a few weeks to a few months before the body gets rid of it. Unlike hepatitis C, it does not become chronic. In 80 percent of cases, untreated chronic hepatitis C, on the other hand, lasts until the person dies of the disease or of some other cause.

The 20 percent who contract only the acute form of hepatitis C get rid of the virus quickly. They may feel a heavy, flu-like sickness within a few weeks after they are infected. They may feel extremely fatigued, lose their appetite, suffer from joint and stomach pains, become nauseous, run a high fever, have a headache, and notice their skin and eyes becoming yellow. The symptoms commonly last from two to twelve weeks. For most people, symptoms may be slight or unnoticeable. In less than six months—the time span that is designated as acute hepatitis C—the virus will be gone from their system.

The chronic stage of hepatitis C hangs around. After decades, people with chronic hep C may experience the same type of symptoms as the few who get sick during the acute stage of the disease. Amazingly, even when the liver begins to stiffen with cirrhosis, many people have no symptoms at all. But eventually, physical effects can emerge. After a while the skin may become itchy. A person with chronic hepatitis C may bruise easily, bleed easily, or acquire spider-like blood vessels on their skin. Swelling in the legs, confusion, or weight loss may occur. These are all signs that cirrhosis is present and the liver is unable to manage all of the jobs in the body that it normally does. But for decades most people with chronic hepatitis C feel fine. It can be an exceedingly long time before those who contract it learn they have it.

Take what happened to Jim Banta, who didn't notice symptoms until nearly thirty years after he was infected. I talked with Jim a year after he was cured. He was sixty-one, but his chipper voice made him sound much younger.

Jim grew up in New York City and in the late 1960s attended Jamaica High School in Queens, about fifty minutes by transit from where I lived at the time. In the summer, I often took a bus to Jamaica with groupie friends. We would alight at a grungy bus stop and scurry with our beach bags to Jamaica Station, where we would board a train to Rockaway Beach. My mother cautioned me to never wander into the side streets near the station, where uncollected litter lay in heaps and old men sat on sidewalks, guzzling brown bottles of brew. "Someone might kidnap you," my mother said.

The area got better as it approached Jim's street, but not by much. He lived in an apartment building near the Hillside Avenue subway station with his parents and three older brothers.

Jim says he was a "hooligan" in high school and had little interest in his studies. He and his buddies would hang around in a local park, smoking and trying to pick up girls. Jim didn't have much problem attracting them. With brown hair streaming past his shoulders, he resembled the comic-strip hero Prince Valiant. He says he and his friends were into defying everything. "That was the sign of the times. Lots of protest going on, and things of that nature," he said. He smoked tobacco, drank beer, and sampled illegal substances. Jim should have graduated from high school in 1972, but his "bad-boy hippie" lifestyle and a family tragedy set him on a different course.

When Jim was seventeen, his second oldest brother, Billy, eight years his elder, was hanging around in Manhattan's Lower East Side. Billy associated with the wrong people, Jim said. "There was an argument and instead of settling it with fists, the guy shot him." Devastated by the murder, Jim quit high school and began injecting drugs. "I injected pretty much everything. Heroin was kind of my drug of choice," he said. "It was bad times." He stuck out his thumb and rode as far from New York City as he could. He made it to Whitehorse in Yukon.

He continued hitchhiking for a couple of years and in 1976 settled in San Francisco. By that time he had contracted hepatitis C. A quarter of a century passed before he knew it.

For most of his adult life Jim lived a happy, stable existence in San Francisco with his wife and two sons. He worked for thirty-five years in the construction industry and has been married for more than thirty.

In the late summer of 2000, Jim was framing an elevator shed at the top of an apartment building. The heat of the day made him sweat and affected his ability to focus. He took a misstep and fell eight feet off the scaffolding. A workmate drove him to the hospital. Jim arrived home with two broken ribs and a football-sized bruise on his right rib cage, which covers the largest lobe of the liver. He felt pain in the area but didn't worry right away. Broken ribs take weeks to heal. Doctors seldom put them in a cast because that could cause breathing problems. Many of the ribs cover the liver, so a pain in the ribs and pain in the liver can feel similar. Jim was hurting, like anyone who had cracked their ribs would be.

His ribs began to heal but about a month later he threw up blood. He thought it was related to the accident, so he returned to the San Francisco General Hospital, where Workers' Compensation had taken care of him. By the time he got there he had lost about half of his blood. He was rushed to intensive care and given a transfusion. As a matter of routine, the hospital tested his blood. The doctors told him he had hepatitis C. And that wasn't the worst of it—he also had end-stage liver disease.

The demon is usually insidious. It can be dormant and then suddenly advance. The 80 percent of people who develop the chronic form of hepatitis C are commonly symptom free for a long, long time. When they first learn they have antibodies, they may feel healthy. That makes it easy for them to think that their disease probably vanished a month or two after they contracted it. Many years later they may be blindsided by the diagnosis. They feel their luck has turned bad, which primes their mind for disaster.

Dr. Radev said if my hep had disappeared during the acute stage, I would have developed antibodies to protect against the disease for the rest of my life. But there's no guaranteed immunity. In a 2010 study of drug users who had cleared acute hepatitis C, researchers at Johns Hopkins Medical Institutions in Baltimore discovered that reinfection is possible. Reinfected individuals are more likely to clear the infection during the acute stage of hepatitis C than to develop the chronic disease. More definitive studies showed similar results with chimpanzees. (Reinfection was easier to prove with chimps because they could be injected with the virus. That was unthinkable with humans—but it was cruel to the chimps.) Nonetheless, people who experience only acute hep C are in luck. If they stay away from contaminated blood, their hepatitis will be gone forever, and so will the viral threat of liver damage.

Chronic hep C can progressively destroy the liver. Like me, most people with the chronic illness may not know what's happening until the destruction is well underway. Brent Fitzsimmons, who runs a harm-reduction needle exchange program on the Sunshine Coast of British Columbia, sees a lot of people with chronic hepatitis C. He says the lack of pain in the early years of the disease is why the virus is rampant among injection drug users. Most of them notice no symptoms. They shoot the virus into their veins with hep-tainted needles and, unaware that they harbor the disease, deliver it to friends who share their needles. "Hepatitis C hides in their system," he said as we chatted on the phone soon after my diagnosis. "People don't often see the doctor until a chance occurrence like yours happens."

Yes, chance revealed the virus to me. I had taken a chance and changed doctors because I didn't like driving long distances. It was by chance that my friend Jen had read about a new doctor in the *Coast Reporter,* and chance had it that Dr. Radev was one of the minority of general practitioners who routinely test for hep. But chance can lead to lucky or unlucky outcomes. I was lucky that I had followed Jen's advice and sought out a new doctor. But as I heard Dr. Radev's diagnosis, I felt immensely unlucky. I felt as if the reality I had always imagined to be true had been a physiological lie. I felt that my attempts to be healthy over my adult life had been useless because of this demon disease. What good were all the fresh veggies I had eaten? What good were all the hikes, yoga, and sit-ups? Nothing had stopped this disease. My mind drifted through a phantom cloud as the doctor spoke. I struggled to come out of it. "Hepatitis C hardens the liver," I heard her say, as I forced myself to pay attention. "It can lead to cirrhosis of the liver or liver cancer."

"Will that happen to me?"

"It usually takes decades," she said.

"I've had it for decades," I said. "I must have gotten it from the blood transfusion."

"You didn't tell me you had a transfusion," she said, seeming puzzled.

I realized I should have been more specific with my doctor. She had asked earlier if I had undergone surgery, and

I had said "no." I think doctors may equate transfusions with surgery or assume they are connected. Mine almost was. After my hemorrhage at the Jewish General Hospital, surgeons debated whether to operate on me. Frequently, a postpartum hemorrhage is followed by surgery—a D&C (dilation and curettage), which cleans out the uterus. The doctors monitored my vitals for several days. I languished in a darkened ward, desperately missing Della and my new baby. Finally, the doctors decided against the surgery. I went home to bond with Jessica.

"I had a transfusion after a postpartum hemorrhage more than forty years ago," I explained to Dr. Radev.

Most studies of the effects of hepatitis C cover up to thirty years, and forty years of chronic hep is rare in the literature. Researchers commonly state that symptoms may not appear for ten, twenty, or thirty years. The demon had swished through my system at least since the early 1970s, and I had yet to definitively feel its effects.

I did have joint pain, my brain seemed foggy, and I had itching—all symptoms of the disease. I had also lost a lot of weight—another symptom. But these things are hard to measure and to directly connect with hep C. My joints had been torn in a car accident, my brain may have been foggy from stress and sleeplessness, the itching in my legs could have come from any number of little sea creatures I regularly wade through at the beach. The weight loss? I had been trying to exercise a lot and to eat non-fattening food.

For most people, chronic hepatitis C hides in their system without any symptoms. But before symptoms appear, there may be signs of the disease. The difference between a "symptom" and a "sign" is that patients experience *symptoms* of disease, while tests reveal *signs* of the disease. Generally, in most diseases, a patient first reports a symptom to a doctor, which leads the doctor to search for signs. In a simplified example, a person may be tired and unusually thirsty. The doctor tests their glucose and discovers a high level of blood sugar. Tiredness and thirst are symptoms of diabetes; a high level of blood sugar is a sign of the disease.

Chronic hepatitis C is likely to produce signs that a doctor can detect well before the patient perceives any symptoms. However, not all signs are definitive. Bill Demish, a retired air traffic controller, learned that many years after he was infected with hep through a blood transfusion. I talked with Bill on the phone and over Skype toward the end of my treatment for hep. He explained that his job required a thorough annual physical. In one such exam, his doctor detected high bilirubin in his blood. The liver creates bilirubin when it breaks down red blood cells, which a normal liver redirects into the stools. With liver disease, excess bilirubin in the blood causes jaundice. Bill was healthy in every other way, so his doctor wasn't concerned.

In another yearly exam, Bill's doctor discovered his ALT levels were high. ALT is an enzyme found mainly in liver cells. It can seep into the bloodstream from a damaged liver. Although a high level of ALT in the blood can be a sign of hepatitis C, it can also indicate other problems, such as mononucleosis, alcoholism, or cancer. "He (my doctor) was kind of concerned," Bill said. "He was thinking cancer, but it turned out it wasn't." It was many more years before the government sent Bill a letter advising him to be tested for hepatitis C. He then learned he was infected. Eventually—and after treatment with interferon—his liver disease advanced into cirrhosis.

When I was infected, there was no way to detect hepatitis C in blood. The disease itself had yet to be discovered.

In 1986 it became possible to protect against HCV in the blood supply. Although scientists did not actually discover the virus until 1989, surrogate testing (a test for elevated liver enzymes in the blood) could indicate non-A, non-B hepatitis.

The disease hepatitis C was found to be a distinct virus in 1989, and the next year a viral test was available. Until the early '90s, blood wasn't always screened. In 1998 a group of people who had acquired hep C from untested blood between 1986 and 1990 launched a class action lawsuit against the Canadian government and the Canadian Red Cross. Bill Demish was one of those who had received untested blood, and decades later he participated in the lawsuit.

Blood screening became pervasive in Canada by 1992. Following recommendations in the Krever Report, which implicated the Canadian Red Cross for mismanaging Canada's blood supply, Canadian Blood Services was formed in 1998 to oversee the country's blood banking system. Understandably and thankfully, CBS, like the American Red Cross, is incredibly cautious about screening blood.

When a donor gives blood, the agency takes several samples for blood typing and for testing for infectious diseases. The tests include nucleic acid amplification testing (NAAT) for hepatitis C. A donor's sample is pooled with other samples. If the pool tests positive for HCV, then the samples are placed into smaller collections and tested again. The tests go on until the infected sample is found. NAAT replicates the virus's genetic material more than a million-fold. This can detect the hep C virus well before antibodies show up in the blood. When I was writing this book, the test was becoming the standard in blood and plasma collection throughout the world. Unfortunately, Bill's transfusion occurred too early.

In late 1986, Bill was working at the Medicine Hat Airport as a flight service specialist. Because Medicine Hat is a small airport, Bill's job encompassed several duties. He scanned the skies and radar to direct air traffic, handled weather briefings, and advised new pilots on flight planning and regulations. If an aircraft strayed from its flight plan, it was Bill's job to investigate.

Once a week after work he and his buddies would play a friendly game of hockey at the local arena. Like most middle-aged but well-toned hockey players, he would take some falls. Normally he would get back up and skate like a firebrand.

One evening he made what he called a "suicide pass." Commanding the puck, Bill sliced through the ice on the way to the goal. Guys from the other team were coming up fast. In a snap second, Bill whizzed by another player and passed the puck to a teammate. He turned his back, spinning sideways. A friend clipped his skates. Bill flew into the air like a missile. He hadn't seen the collision coming, so he couldn't protect himself as he landed. He smacked onto the ice, whacking his back. He lay stunned on the cold, hard surface. For a second he didn't know what had happened. His team members gathered around, ready to help him, but before they could pull him up, he stumbled off the ice. After a while he returned for another shift. He lunged ahead with his stick. Suddenly pain wracked his body. His mind blurred. "Oh, God, I can't do this," he told himself. He retreated to the boards. "Bingo. That was it," he said when I spoke with him.

Bill managed to drive home and take a shower. As water streamed down, his mind cleared enough to focus on his duty at the airport. It was almost the beginning of the graveyard shift, and he had to replace a co-worker who had already put in a long day of sky watching. It was a critical position that could not be left empty. Bill drummed up his stamina and drove to work. He trembled as he climbed up the two flights of stairs to the observation tower. As he gazed through an expanse of glass toward the runway, chills spread through his body and he began to shake. "I can't stay here," he told his co-worker. The man wanted to leave, so Bill called a woman who liked working nights. She arrived to cover his shift, and he left.

Bill steeled himself once again and drove to the Medicine Hat hospital's emergency department. A doctor checked him over, gave him two aspirins, and sent him home. "That was the worst thing to do," Bill said. At home again, he was in agony. His son, who was on winter break from university, insisted that he drive Bill to the hospital. The son sped through town with his father barely conscious. They arrived at the hospital between 3 and 4 a.m.

Bill's son asked for the doctor who had treated his father earlier. "He gave the doctor hell," Bill recalls. The doctor immediately called in a surgeon. Within two hours, Bill was under anesthesia. Beneath glaring lights, a surgery team sliced open his torso.

They discovered he had been bleeding internally around his stomach. Blood had congealed in his kidneys, which ceased to function. As doctors repaired the organs, they pumped fifteen units of blood into Bill. He awoke on New Year's Eve in the intensive care unit. The staff was celebrating, making the ward "noisy as hell," which wasn't the best atmosphere for recovery. Nonetheless, within a few days Bill's kidneys were okay. He didn't know that hepatitis C had entered his body through unscreened blood he received during the surgery. "I believe they got it from some jail in Arkansas," Bill said in his gruff, grandfatherly voice.

He discovered the nefarious origin of the blood some fifteen years later, after he had retired from the airport job. He got a letter from the Alberta government in 2001 that suggested he get an antigen test. He had blood taken and learned he had been infected with hepatitis C.

Bill wasn't overly concerned at first because he didn't know much about the disease. "I thought, well, the buggers gave me bad blood," he said. "It ticked me off a little bit, but I didn't get overexcited about it." Hep C was in the news a lot in those days because of the lawsuit. "There was quite a flap over it," Bill says. Nonetheless, he thought the disease was temporary, something he would shake off on his own.

One of his two sons had come down with hepatitis A years before and gradually and fully recovered. Bill at first thought hepatitis C was much like that.

When he learned the differences between the two discrete diseases, his complacency vanished. His doctor sent him to a specialist, who put him on interferon for six months. At the end of that time, the virus was undetectable. But six months later, Bill learned that some hepatitis C RNA had remained in his system, hidden. The disease was back. Interferon at that time was commonly combined with ribavirin, which was considered the most effective treatment, yet he had received only shots of interferon. Bill now thinks the specialist "screwed up." Although it's possible the doctor had prescribed the correct treatment, "maybe he didn't monitor the thing property," Bill said, suggesting that he himself either did not receive or did not take ribavirin.

Next his general practitioner referred him to a hepatology clinic in Calgary. Bill was put on a waiting list, and it was close to a year before he got an appointment. "That would have taken longer, except my son was in Calgary, pounding on their door," he said.

A specialist at the Calgary Hepatology Clinic said Bill should have been taking Pegasys (interferon), plus Copegus 200 mg tablets (ribavirin). He put Bill on both for a one-year treatment. "They finally got their act together," Bill said. "I think, if I had gotten in there right away, I never would have got the cirrhosis." According to a biopsy performed between his two treatments, Bill's liver damage had become serious. There is no specific time span needed for the liver to harden into cirrhosis, but aging is known to hasten the process.

The first treatment had made Bill weak, nauseated, and tired, and the second treatment was far worse. "It got to the point where I could barely crawl up the stairs," he recalled. "My wife said I was miserable." On top of that, his daughter-in-law was dying, so Bill and his wife went back and forth to Grande Prairie—ten hours away by car—to visit her. Bill often thought of quitting the drugs, but he persevered. After six months he noticed his heart rate had gone "out of whack," often missing beats. "I got hold of Calgary and immediately they said, 'Get off that stuff.'" Nonetheless, Bill praised the doctor and staff at the Calgary clinic for their high standard of care. After that partial second treatment, he was clear of the virus, and he stayed that way.

WHEN HEP C ATTACKS, infected cells band together, thicken, and form scars; this scarring is called *fibrosis.* The liver progressively hardens. While there is still enough healthy liver tissue for the organ to function normally, the scars later become so tight that the liver becomes like bumpy leather. This is called *cirrhosis,* and it moves from *compensated cirrhosis* through *decompensated cirrhosis.* In the compensated stage, the liver is heavily scarred but functioning. Patients are likely to experience few symptoms or none at all. So hep C can continue to hide, even at this dangerous stage. In decompensated cirrhosis, symptoms rear up and become progressively more pronounced. They can begin much like acute hep C symptoms but get worse. A long list of other symptoms may appear, such as swollen legs and enlarged veins in the esophagus.

In all, 20 to 25 percent of people with chronic hepatitis C develop cirrhosis in twenty to twenty-five years. Beyond that, the rate increases. Untreated, 4 percent of those who develop cirrhosis will end up with liver cancer. After my first visit with the gastroenterologist who treated my hepatitis, I learned I may have been at the compensated stage. The Phantom Zone became cloudier and darker. I wished that Superman would save me.

## 1968 and 1970

# DRUGGIES

I MET MANNY in New York City at a loft party when I was still with Kevin. Among the crowded gathering of musicians and actors, Manny stood out because of his height. He was about the same height as Kevin, who was six foot three.

Manny had black wavy hair past his ears and a well-trimmed mustache, and his eyes were a deep ocean blue. I introduced him to Kevin, and he soon became one of the small bunch of friends Kevin and I had in common. When I left Kevin, I lost track of Manny.

Some two years later, I was living in Montreal. Peter and I had found a large, run-down apartment near McGill University. We decided to beautify the plywood kitchen floor by gluing down a checkerboard of black and white tiles. Goldberry, our cat, raced into the kitchen and galloped through the glue tray. Her paws left stringy, sticky trails. I felt weak, but I grabbed her. "*Meeee-yeemeeee*," she yowled. As she scratched to get away from me, I managed to douse her feet with turpentine. Then I slumped to the floor, exhausted. After that I couldn't get up. I crawled away from the tile job, thinking I had been poisoned by fumes. But I wasn't. It seemed to be the beginning of the flu. Within a few hours, Peter had succumbed to the bug as well. We spent the next three days moaning, sleeping, heaving, and eating nothing. Was the glue scene with the cat really the beginning of the flu? I wondered many years later. Maybe it was hep.

One day, while stepping onto the short set of stairs up to that Montreal apartment, I slipped on ice. As I tumbled backward, a man caught my arm.

"Thank you!" I looked up at the tall, clean-cut man. Something seemed odd.

"No problem. Are you okay? Hey, don't I know you?"

I stared at him quizzically.

"It's me, Manny."

"Manny? Oh, Manny! What are you doing here?" I scanned his face. It was the same face I remembered, without the mustache, but his cheeks were hollow. He had been thin before, but now he was gaunt.

"I've been living in Montreal awhile," Manny said.

"Why don't you come up to my place?" I said. "It's right here." I pointed at the door five steps up.

In the freshly floored kitchen, Manny told Peter, "I'm selling pot. If you want any you should come by soon. I'm applying for a job, and if I get it, I'll be getting rid of my stash."

One night we got a babysitter and visited Manny at his apartment, where he lived with his girlfriend, Kim, an office assistant. "Did you find a job?" I asked Manny as he weighed dark green leaves on a balance scale. Seeds rolled off the balance plate. In those days, when you bought marijuana, the seeds came along as well.

"I almost got a job as a cop," Manny said. "I passed all the tests. But then they weighed me. They said I was too thin."

We commiserated with him and invited Manny and Kim to a cottage we would be visiting soon. It was a friend's family's vacation home on a lake in the Eastern Townships, and we had been told we could bring other guests. Our friend Janice's mother owned the cottage. Six adults plus my daughter would be going, and now there would be eight. Janice had assured us the place was more than large enough.

The day after we all arrived at the charming log home on the sparkling, cold lake, Manny and Kim skipped dinner, saying they were ill. The next day they got sicker. They said they couldn't leave their room. Janice and I took turns knocking on their door, asking if they wanted anything. Kim would squeak, "No." The following day, Manny and Kim started yelling at each other. Sounds of banging objects came from the room. I also heard retching, and when I went near the door I smelled vomit.

The six adults outside of that bedroom convened a meeting. I suggested that Manny and Kim had caught the cat glue flu. I went to the door and asked whether they wanted us to call a doctor. "No!" Kim screamed.

The next morning Janice said, "This is my mother's place. I can't have some horrible disease infecting it. I'm going to talk with them and call a doctor." She barged through the door and stayed in the room fifteen minutes.

She came out shaking her head and raking her curly hair with her fingers. "They're junkies," she said. "They didn't bring any heroin."

Many people hold a stereotype of depraved, criminally nasty heroin users. But Manny and Kim were nice people. I would have never known they were addicts if they hadn't gone cold turkey in my presence. And though a lot of people have contracted hepatitis C through the use of intravenous drugs, many of them used a needle only once or twice. Still, those who dabble with IV drugs are playing chicken with hepatitis C. After blood screening became the norm in the 1990s, IV drug use supplanted transfusions in creating the highest risk for the disease in the developed world. According to a 2016 study from the Public Health Agency of Canada, among people infected with HCV who have no other risk factors, 61 percent have reported using intravenous drugs.

Yet some IV drug users stay free from HCV. If an uninfected drug user never shares a needle with someone else who has the disease, there will be no virus to pass along. That's why safe injection programs are important.

As for Manny, I never heard from him again. I hope that was only because he was embarrassed about the scene at the cottage. I hope he and Kim kicked their heroin habit. I hope they never contracted hepatitis C.

# PART II

*MANIFESTATION*

## CHAPTER 5

# STIGMA AND SHARING

T HE DAY SHE told me I had hep, Dr. Radev warned that I could easily get sick from something else. While the immune system is combating HCV, it has less strength to fend off other pathogens. And if the body is attacked by a different virus, the blood might launch an all-out battle against the new invader, leaving fewer resources to fight hepatitis C. I had been living with hepatitis C for forty years, and compared with my family and friends, I felt I had succumbed to just slightly more than a normal number of viruses for that time period—and most of them had been colds. That, along with my penchant for healthy eating and exercise, made me think I had a better-than-average immune system. I may have lost the early fight against HCV by only a hair. That was just my luck—bad luck on the one side, but great luck compared with those who had to endure a more complicated illness.

People who are coinfected with HCV and HIV, for example, must deal with a severely compromised immune system. The human immunodeficiency virus and hepatitis C are both RNA viruses, but unlike the virus that causes AIDS, hepatitis C does not infect immune cells. The hepatitis C virus invades liver cells and turns them into its own virus factories, but the blood system can still produce antibodies against other diseases. HIV/AIDS infects and destroys the blood's T-helper white blood cells, where it reproduces and stops the production of antibodies. Unfortunately, 25 percent of people infected with HIV are also infected with hepatitis C.

Ben Handley and Dennis Ronson are a devoted long-time couple who found themselves in that predicament. I visited them in Victoria, British Columbia, not long after my diagnosis. On a hot day under a crystal blue sky, Ben and I lounged at a patio table overlooking his swimming pool and expansive gardens. A Fallopia vine, thick with white flowers, hung over a trellis that fenced off the pool. Zinnias, hibiscus, and rhododendrons surrounded us with color. Ben brought me a glass of water, which is at the top of my list of liver-healthy beverages.

Ben's curly gray hair framed a deeply weathered face and a chin covered with gray-brown stubble. His hazel eyes glinted in the sun. At sixty-four he saw himself continuing to work as a sociology professor far into the future. He said he loves teaching, research, and traveling the world to speak at conferences about social issues. But because he was infected with both hepatitis C and HIV, he'd had to take a break from his job for eleven years.

He learned about the HIV more than a decade earlier. Then a blood test that was part of his HIV testing revealed he had hep. He wracked his brain and couldn't figure out how he had contracted hepatitis C. Regardless, he wanted to get rid of it so that he would have only one disease to deal with. Ben's liver was just moderately damaged, but the doctor—a specialist in both infections—wanted him to get as well as possible so that he could take care of his HIV. In November 2008 Ben began months of treatment with ribavirin and injected interferon. The side effects—both physical and emotional—were horrible, he said. Meanwhile, Ben learned that Dennis, his cherished companion, was also coinfected. The interferon didn't work for Ben, and he worried about his partner. Ben had built an exemplary career and a pastoral setting for his home, but his illnesses had cost him his peace of mind.

I had zero risk factors for HIV, but I thought about other illnesses that might threaten me. Dr. Radev was particularly concerned about hepatitis B, which could double the attack on my liver. Between my diagnosis and the date of my first appointment with a gastroenterologist, she sent me to a local clinic for vaccinations. She also ordered an ultrasound of my liver. "We should hurry with that," she said.

In the months following my diagnosis, I visited the public health clinic in Gibsons three times and received a series of shots for tetanus, diphtheria, pneumococcus, and hepatitis B.

My blood tests had turned up antibodies for hepatitis A, so Dr. Radev asked if I had ever been ill with it. "No," I said, puzzled. I thought back to Peter, who had turned yellow after working in a restaurant in the Caribbean. Maybe I had picked up hep A from him, not noticed symptoms, and shaken it off. Then I realized the source of the antibodies. In 2004 I had gone to Trinidad and Tobago to attend a wedding and write a magazine story. I had been vaccinated against hepatitis A before I left.

DURING MY FIRST appointment at the vaccination clinic, I talked with the nurse about my disease. She was pleasant and sympathetic, but she didn't mince words about the possible outcomes of hep: cirrhosis, cancer, or both. Until I could be treated and cured I needed to do everything I could to make sure I didn't succumb to some other malevolent pathogen. She assumed I would be treated with interferon— not much was publicly known about other treatments then—and she commiserated with me about the painful injections and side effects. At the time, even the new drugs Dr. Radev mentioned would have to be taken with interferon. A benefit of the new, direct-acting antivirals was that they would reduce the number of weeks interferon was needed.

One of interferon's most common side effects is severe, frequent nausea. In the past I had suffered through three terrible bouts of flu, including the sickness that hit when my cat ran through glue. All three times, I had wanted to die rather than wallow in another minute of stomach agony. Interferon was almost guaranteed to be worse. I was sure I would give up the drug before I was cured. That meant, at that time, that I would probably never be cured. That meant, at that time, that my liver damage would have a good chance of getting worse.

Interferon is actually a natural cytokine protein, which is manufactured by the human body. Cytokines trigger the immune system to attack viruses. Interferon interferes with viral replication, hence its name.

In the 1990s people being treated for hepatitis C had to inject interferon two or three times a week. In 2001, Roche came out with peginterferon alfa-2a (pegylated interferon, brand name Pegasys), which stays in the system longer. Patients only had to inject the drug once a week. But the side effects were the same.

Ben Handley recalled getting Pegasys injections, which were paired with ribavirin, an antiviral drug that suppressed replication of HCV in the body. Ben started treatment with injected interferon and with ribavirin tablets in November 2008. The physical and emotional effects were wretched. Within two months he had developed anemia (a common effect of ribavirin) and lost about eighteen pounds. He had always been a fitness buff but no longer had the strength to work out at the gym. He would spend all day trying to eat. After a simple breakfast he would become violently nauseated. He'd rest awhile, try to chew and swallow something else, and get sick again. After about three hours he could sometimes keep down a piece of toast.

He couldn't walk up the stairs in his spacious two-level home. He would pull a few weeds in the garden and collapse on the grass. He was becoming depressed, not only from frustration, but also from the Pegasys, which lists depression as a common side effect.

Nonetheless, Ben felt supported by his friends and his partner throughout the ordeal. His spouse, Dennis, administered the injections. Interferon must be injected into fat; it can't go into muscle. Ben was so lean that Dennis had to push the syringe into his back, where there were fat deposits. The injections were painful, and Dennis moved them each week to the opposite side of Ben's back to prevent scarring. He did so for an extremely cranky partner.

"It was an emotional roller-coaster ride," Ben said, and Dennis got the brunt of it. "I'd be hysterical laughing one minute and bawling my eyes out the next. I kept saying to him, you're going to leave me. I know you're going to leave me." But Dennis, healthy and athletic-looking despite having the same coinfection, hung on.

Ben endured the treatment for almost seven months. He recalled a conversation with his doctor:

"How are you doing?" the doctor said.

Ben described his depression and physical weakness.

"You're not in the hospital, are you? You're not hooked up to an IV that's replenishing your blood. Is there anything we can do so you can keep on?" the doctor asked. "Because you may not have cleared the virus yet."

"If I have to try again sometime in the future, I'll have to do that because I can't do it anymore now," Ben said, and with that he abandoned the hep meds.

Stories like that ramped up my fear. I was a wimp when it came to stomach troubles. I would never be able to handle any treatment that contained interferon, which, at that time, all treatments except some specious herbal remedies did. If I were to give up on treatment, I would never get rid of the hep. But if those demons were to stay in my liver, I believed I would be a sure goner.

I would think these self-defeating thoughts while listening to friends chatting about housing prices or their new Sheltie puppy. I struggled to maintain a semblance that I was paying attention without giving my secret away. Yet I yearned to have a sounding board that didn't involve my family, who worried too much about me already. I took the ferry to North Vancouver twice a week for work and couldn't avoid talking with colleagues. In the work setting I felt even more reticent. I worried that if I revealed my infection to workmates, they would think I was strange, dirty, or ultra-contagious. They might inadvertently send gossip up the administrative chain. The higher-ups might think I was contagious too. After all, before I learned I had hep, I had hardly known anything about the disease. In the past I too would have thought it was easily transmissible.

My apprehension turned out to be true—with a few people among many. Two of my friends seemed to avoid me once they heard of my illness. They became just occasional acquaintances. I lost communication with a family member. And I believe I lost one person's friendship entirely when I talked with her about my disease.

I had lunch with Ellen less than three weeks post-diagnosis. Ellen and I had worked together as volunteers in a writers' organization more than twenty years before and had managed an event together. We had remained fast but occasional friends. Ellen would nudge me four or five times a year, and we'd meet in a restaurant or pub. Once or twice a year we'd see a movie together.

I had set up the lunch with her three weeks earlier, a day or two before my diagnosis. We sat across from each other at the Vancouver Art Gallery's outdoor café, which overlooks touristy Robson Square.

As we ate, Ellen expounded on her coming trek in Spain, yet I heard her with just about a fifth of my brain. The other four-fifths was fixated on my impending misery. My mind was running a loop, twirling through the choice of dying from liver disease or spending a year running back and forth to the bathroom, throwing up. I also kept trying to think of a way to tell Ellen I had hep.

"My mom's been ill," she said, as she cut into the cheese-filled quesadilla on her plate.

"Oh no. That's too bad. What's wrong?" I asked, thinking whatever illness her mother had was probably not as bad as hepatitis C. I thought I could squeeze in a mention of my disease and finally let it out in the open, at least with this one friend.

"A stroke. But she's recovering," she said.

A stroke is serious, I thought, and it's more likely to kill

39065140363407

# Viorel,
# Sandra

Pickup By: December 14,
2017

you than hepatitis C. But her mother was recovering. "It's good that she's getting better," I said. Ellen talked about her mother's situation, and I asked questions about it.

As we finished our lunches and each ordered pie à la mode, the conversation segued into the usefulness of living close to downtown, the good fortune of living near a hospital, Ellen's recent visit to the hospital for a pelvic ultrasound, and, finally, the recent ultrasound of my liver. Once the pies arrived and the server had left the table, I threw in, "I just learned I have hepatitis C."

"Oh. Oh, really?" Ellen said.

"Yes."

I told her about my blood transfusion and how I had acquired a new doctor who had discovered the hep. Ellen stared directly at her apple pie as I talked, not once looking up. She pushed around pieces of crust with her fork, mushing them into the ice cream. Then she pushed the half-eaten pie away. She moved her chair back from the table and looked at me, just a bit. "I've got to get back to work. We should get the check," she said.

We paid. We left the restaurant. "Gotta go," she said, avoiding our usual hug. Two days later I emailed Ellen saying lunch had been fun, and it was too bad she didn't have more time off from work. I invited her to my home. Even though Ellen used to email or call me once a month or so, I never heard back—even after I emailed her again, twice. I surmised she was afraid of catching hep.

I TALKED ABOUT people's fear of contagion with Bill Demish, the air traffic controller who was injured in a hockey game. He asked me, "Did you notice that when people found out you had hep C, there was a bit of treating you like a leper?"

"Yes, I noticed," I said. I thought about Ellen's body language as she picked at the pie. I asked Bill what he does when the stigma rears up at him. He explained his philosophy with an example.

One day, he said, he was in Grande Prairie, Alberta, having coffee with a friend. He told his friend about his hep. After Bill went home, his wife said his friend had called and asked, "Gee. Should I be worried about this?"

Bill said his friend may have been worrying whether he might have caught hep from Bill in the coffee shop, but more likely he was thinking back to all of his interactions with Bill, not knowing if the hepatitis virus could jump from person to person in a handshake or be sprinkled into the air with a sneeze.

"I definitely felt some of my friends kind of back away," Bill told me. "A lot of people thought hep was about the same as AIDS, and there was more stigma with AIDS than there should have been." Bill said it wasn't worth worrying much about the stigma. When people hear you have hep, they eventually get used to it, he said.

But before they do, awkward and disheartening moments can arise. John Lavette, the retired flower merchant, said when he first tells friends about his infection, he almost hears them thinking, "Get away from me. I don't want it. You're going to give me something shitty." He doesn't blame these people, he said. They may just be ignorant. But when he explains his disease to a person a second time, sometimes "they're still freaky about it, and they try to avoid you." That's not fair, he says. He didn't ask for his disease.

Neither did I. Neither did anyone.

After the lunch with Ellen, I tended to suss people out for many weeks before I would decide whether to reveal that I had hep. Daryl Luster, president of the Pacific

Hepatitis C Network, said he fell into a similar pattern. As we chatted in a Starbucks in Richmond, British Columbia, he said he had been sick with symptoms for three years before he was diagnosed. When he finally learned he had hepatitis C, it took him two months to tell anyone outside of his family. Once he began to talk with them about his disease, he noticed he had two levels of friendships. There were genuine friends who showed empathy, but others seemed oblivious to his feelings and began to treat him "as if my breath were contagious," he said. He said he dropped those "second-tier" friends from his circle.

Despite that setback so common to people with hepatitis C, Daryl ultimately opened up to everyone who would listen to him. He now works with the Pacific Hepatitis C Network and speaks to audiences all over the world as an advocate for people with hepatitis C. He said one of the things that changed him was that while he was being treated with interferon, his dad was dying of kidney cancer. It was the last six months of his dad's life. Daryl visited him often at the hospital. "Looking back, it was the most difficult time of my life but in some ways it was a beautiful time because I chose to look at it in a different light. He was more worried about me than about himself, and of course I was more worried about him than about myself."

That became the approach that worked for me. At the time I was diagnosed with hep, two of my friends had been undergoing chemo for breast cancer. After the experience with Ellen, I met each of them separately for coffee. They were both gracious and courageous. Despite the travails of their own serious condition, they listened to my worries about hepatitis C. They seemed more concerned about me than about themselves, like Daryl had been with his dad. I began to feel more confident about revealing my illness. Still,

I wasn't ready to fully emerge from my shell with just anyone, so I went to see my friend Nita, who herself had hep.

Several years back, Nita had been cruising on her motorcycle straight along the inside lane of a busy street in Vancouver. A car on the right crossed her path, trying to turn left. Nita couldn't stop the motorcycle. She bounced over the front of her bike and slammed into the back of the car, catching her ankle on the car's rear bumper. The bumper flew off, pulling her with it across the pavement. She was dazed at first; then she checked the painful spots. Gashes covered her arm and leg. A bumper screw stuck out through the skin of her ankle, which was fractured and throbbing.

As an ambulance sped off with her inside, she told the paramedics: "I know my name. I know what day it is. I know where I am. I don't want a tetanus shot or any painkillers." At the hospital, a nurse cut off Nita's blood-sticky clothes and ran a saline drip into her arm for rehydration. When the nurse left, Nita ripped out the IV. She stumbled out of the hospital and hobbled down to the street in a hospital gown.

"I was in a major amount of pain," she recalled as we chatted in the living room of the open-plan condo she had just bought. "I sat on a stool in the tub and ran hot and cold water, on and off, on and off, over my ankle for ten minutes at a time. I elevated my ankle, and I'd massage it and sing to it." After a few days, she returned to work, hopping into the office on her good right leg.

Just as she rejected hospital care after the accident, Nita has refused to let conventional doctors treat her hepatitis C. Instead of using allopathic medicines, she follows a liver-protective diet. The diet is full of no-no's: no alcohol, no coffee, no refined sugar, no wheat. She eats lots of mangoes, papayas, eggplant, and garlic. Every day for forty-nine days she ate a can of white kidney beans, which she says produce natural interferon. She ingests Chinese remedies, including turmeric and milk thistle—both scientifically shown to protect the liver—and bitter tea. She doesn't use soap and washes her skin with olive oil.

Nita acquired HCV from her mother. In the early 1970s, Nita's parents and two older sisters lived a comfortable life near the beach in Mombasa, Kenya, a city not known for the safest medical practices. There Nita's mother received blood transfusions during pregnancy. HCV seeped into her bloodstream and into the fetus, who was Nita. Mother-to-fetus transmission happens in about 6 percent of pregnancies when the mother has hep, and the risk is higher if the mom has HIV.

The family moved to Canada when Nita was two, and life went on. But in the 1990s Nita's mother began to feel sick. She visited a doctor and was diagnosed with hepatitis C. When I talked with Nita, her mother was seventy-six and had yellowed skin and eyes. She endures frequent nausea and weakness, symptoms of cirrhosis. Nita began experiencing the same symptoms when she was thirty. Twelve years after that, she was almost free of them.

Nita had learned of her infection while working as an editor in a busy production office. She vomited frequently. She felt pain in her upper abdomen, where the liver rests just under the ribs. Her skin had turned sallow. She often took sick days. "I felt like a clock ticking," Nita said. "I had been so sick and was feeling like I was on the edge of hitting rock bottom." In desperation, she spent $300 on a comprehensive blood test. It showed enzyme levels that matched those that occur with hepatitis C. Given her mother's diagnosis and history, Nita knew she had the disease without getting screened for the virus itself.

Today Nita works as a personal trainer at a community center. She has the sinewy body, muscles, and grace you would expect of a woman in her profession. But her porcelain-smooth complexion shows a yellow tint. She said she expects the jaundice to vanish once she has purified herself.

"Do you feel like you're being cured?" I asked.

"There are rough patches, but I feel that things can be regenerated. It's a matter of removing negative thought patterns," she explained. In addition to being meticulous about her diet, Nita is working on calming her consciousness. She steers clear of internalized anger, which creates liver imbalances, she said. To purify her mind, she decorated her condo according to feng shui principles. She led me outside and showed me the cedar floor of her newly renovated deck. It tilts slightly downward to help with energy flow.

Just before I left, she showed me one of her symptoms. The right cheek tends to swell with hepatitis, she said, as she leaned toward me and pointed to the right side of her face. I discerned a little puffiness that I probably wouldn't have noticed on my own.

I left through the patio gate, through a treed path to the parking area. When I got into my car I pulled down the driver's-side visor and gazed into the mirror underneath. I stared at my right cheek. I thought it looked puffy, but it was hard to be sure. Nita had seemed in tune with herself and the universe. Maybe I could slow the progression of my hep with Chinese medicine, or at least use it to soothe my mind. I began researching natural medicines. Among wise and not-so-wise advice, I read about possible non-Western cures from people like Johnny Delirious.

Delirious wrote the book *Hepatitis C, Cured*, which he self-published. At one point, Delirious reveals, his hepatitis C viral load reached 5 million and his doctor said

96 percent of his liver was cirrhotic. Delirious says the doctor who diagnosed him with hepatitis C told him he had only eight months to live.

Delirious grew up in Fort Walton, on the Florida Panhandle, a four-hour drive from New Orleans. He says he caught hep C from eating bad shrimp in Mexico. (Not one of the hundreds of experts and journal articles I researched concurred with that method of transmission.)

Like Nita, Delirious rejected Western medicine. Like Nita, he swore by milk thistle. Studies show that milk thistle can counteract liver damage from substances including Tylenol and death cap mushrooms, and it may help the liver grow new cells. But most other health techniques Delirious employed failed to mesh with medical science—or common sense. Like Nita, Johnny Delirious took up physical training—in his case, kung fu, which could keep his body toned and ready to tackle an infection. But Johnny also tried many spurious methods. He hired an electrician to build a device that zapped him with alternating current at 30,000 cycles per second. For twenty-one days he injected a compound of sodium chloride (salt), ethanol, ammonium chloride, nitrate, and water. He was repeatedly immersed in a hyperbaric oxygen tank (commonly used to treat the bends in deep sea divers). He swallowed megadoses of nutrients. He bought and used a $2,600 oscillating treatment machine. Delirious claims that after his eclectic self-treatment regimen, his viral load sank to zero. The hepatitis antibodies vanished from his blood, he claims. He says that according to his doctor, his cirrhosis-ravaged liver became "the liver of a man in his twenties," though Johnny was fifty-three at the time.

I can't say whether Johnny was actually cured, but I hope he was. Yet I shudder to contemplate the sketchy

treatments some people like Johnny with hep C undergo.[1]
It seems they all want to avoid interferon, and today they
should be able to, if only they can drum up enough cash for
the latest drugs.

On my next visit to Dr. Radev, I asked her about non-
standard approaches to treating hepatitis C. "I've seen a lot
of people who opt for that, and it doesn't work for them,"
Dr. Radev said. She recalled a patient who had a type of
cancer that was completely curable with chemo, but the
patient believed in alternative medicine and refused chemotherapy. "And she died," Dr. Radev said.

But in my opinion, alternative medicine is better than no
medicine because no medicine often equals no hope. While
people wait for treatment, natural methods of improving
liver function may help slow the progress of fibrosis. Misha
Cohen, a member of the San Francisco Hepatitis C Task
Force, firmly believes that. Misha practices "integrated
Chinese medicine," which recognizes the value of Chinese methods and also interacts with Western medicine.
"There's no evidence that Chinese herbs can cure hepatitis,"
she said on the phone. But Chinese methods work well to
give people better health and composure before and after
treatment.

Misha wrote *The Hepatitis C Help Book,* published in
2000. Her coauthor, Dr. Robert Gish, is a clinical professor
of medicine at the Stanford Medical Center and has served
on the editorial boards of several hepatology journals.
When he and Misha wrote the book, interferon treatment
was the norm. Many doctors, like Gish, went to Misha for
help with patients who were experiencing harrowing side
effects.

Misha says she has worked with "many, many, many,
many" people who underwent a long ordeal with interferon.

Chinese medicine improved their health whether the treatment cured them or not, she said. Misha said that under her guidance, some 90 percent of her patients who were taking interferon were able to continue with their entire treatment, and about 85 percent of them cleared the virus. A randomized study in Naples, Italy, found that 27 percent of patients taking interferon and ribavirin for hepatitis C prematurely stopped treatment because of adverse side effects.

In addition, Chinese medicine can stave off the progression of liver disease, Misha said. In the past, that helped delay the need for interferon. In the era of costly direct-acting antiviral drugs, people turn to Chinese medicine to stay healthy while they wait for Medicare, Medicaid, provincial programs, or insurance companies to approve their treatment with direct-acting antivirals. Accessibility of treatment has become a major issue, Misha said.

She guides patients through diet, herbs, and exercise. She admitted that she can't keep everyone's liver disease from progressing to cirrhosis, "but I think we can help a substantial number of people." Her treatment calms people, she said, and added that when someone has just been diagnosed, they may be especially fearful.

I was fearful when I was diagnosed. Like Misha recommends, I modified my diet with liver-healthy foods (see the Appendix). I also gave up a lot of freelance work, which added time for introspection to my days. I thought about the people in my life, those like my husband and daughters, who were helping me face the demon, and others, like Ellen, who made things worse. I thought about the chain of people who had linked my life together, and I looked back into my hippie days when I had likely acquired the virus. Dr. Radev's speculation about sexual transmission kept tapping at my consciousness. According to the Mayo Clinic, sexual transmission of hep C is rare and extremely doubtful in long-term monogamous relationships. The hepatitis C virus carried in someone's blood must seep into another person's bloodstream in order to transmit the infection. HCV RNA has been found in the semen of 18 percent of men who carry the virus and in about double as many men who are coinfected with HIV/AIDS. But semen doesn't normally flow into a partner's blood unless the sex is very rough and produces blood. A study of 500 monogamous, heterosexual couples found that transmission of hepatitis C occurs in only one out of 190,000 sexual encounters.[2] That means that if you have sex with your infected *monogamous* partner every day for 250 years, you would have about a 50–50 chance of catching the virus. I've been with my husband for over 30 years, and I was sure I contracted hep much earlier than that. Al has been tested, and I never passed hep C along to him. According to study after study, the transmission rate among monogamous partners is insignificant. The Centers for Disease Control and Prevention say monogamous couples don't need to use condoms unless one of the partners has HIV/AIDS. But no one with hepatitis C should share razors, toothbrushes, or nail clippers or have unprotected sex during menstruation.

And if you're promiscuous, most sources say, the chances of catching hep C through sex go up. In the hippie era, when I probably acquired the virus, no one talked about promiscuity; they called it free love. "Make love, not war" was the mantra.

John Lavette believed in free love, and he's pretty sure it led to hepatitis C. It happened in the early 1970s, when he hung out in San Francisco's Haight-Ashbury district. Sex with many partners was normal for twenty-something hippies like John. He acknowledges there were risks. "At that age we figured we were invincible," he said. "Every time there was an opportunity to live that lifestyle, we did it."

As a kid in San Francisco, John lived with his grandmother. When she had a day off from her job at Pacific Telephone, she would dress up and take him on the bus downtown. They'd ramble through Chinatown, where they often visited a restaurant on Washington Street. They'd eat cheap Chinese food, and John's grandmother would indulge in one of the restaurant's 50-cent alcoholic drinks. From there they'd stroll to Union Square, where she liked to browse for fashionable clothes at the I. Magnin's store on Geary Street.

"When I'd come out of I. Magnin's I'd see this guy on the corner, and he'd be selling flowers," John said. He was awed and intrigued by the colorful blooms that filled every spot at the flower stand. It was on the corner of one of the busiest places around, and yet to John it seemed like an island of calm within a sea of people and cars. He watched the flower seller happily greet customers, and he figured it would be a great way to make a living. Much, much later, John would become a flower vendor on that very corner. In the meantime, as he grew into his teenage years, John became wild. "I'd get pretty goofy and I'd do stupid stuff," he said.

John's grandmother was concerned. She had taken care of John since he was two. When he was older, her own family had grown, "and now she was saddled with her crazy son's son," John said.

His mother was catatonic and confined to the Napa State Hospital, where she remained for ten years, through many electroshock treatments. John's dad, a seaman, had gone blind in one eye while on a ship to Japan. The other eye continued to deteriorate, and he endured intense, unrelenting pain. In those days the only way to get rid of such pain was morphine. John's dad became addicted to morphine while at sea, and when he arrived back in the States he turned to heroin. He stayed with his son and his mother, John's grandmother, for several years.

At age six or seven, John opened the door of the bathroom and saw his father sitting on the toilet seat next to the sink. His left hand was wrapped around a rubber hose, and he was injecting himself with his right hand. John froze. "Get out of here," his father said.

John has thought about the scene often and remembers every detail. "It was like a photograph," he said.

"To be honest," John said, "he used to use me as a delivery boy." When John was seven his dad enlisted him to make regular visits to a bar in the Tenderloin district, one of the roughest areas of San Francisco. John would walk there by himself, carrying a sandwich bag. "Ostensibly it was for the bartender, for lunch. But there would be balloons of heroin inside."

To John the task was fun. The bartender would lift him onto the bar next to one of those machines with a claw that grabs prizes. John would play and chat with the customers. They would take care of him.

His dad died (possibly with HCV in his liver from drug injections), and John left home at age eighteen. He let his hair grow wild. It didn't fall down his back like the usual hippie hair but flew straight out at the side in the Pacific Islander tradition, which was his heritage. Sometimes it stuck out so wide that when he was lighting a joint, he would accidentally set his hair on fire.

John learned about hepatitis when his cousin came back from Vietnam and passed hepatitis A along to him.

Hep A's symptoms are much the same as those felt in the acute form of hepatitis C. These symptoms may also be felt when chronic hep C becomes advanced:

- Fever
- Nausea and vomiting
- Stomach pain
- Fatigue
- Light-colored stools
- Dark-colored urine
- Joint pain
- Low appetite
- Jaundice

John believes hepatitis C entered his bloodstream between 1966 and 1972. He was doing drugs: LSD, pot, speed, pills—mostly pills. And he wasn't taking care of his body. He figures his immune system was at such a low level that he was easily susceptible to any bug that came his way. Although LSD is not on the list of HCV transmission routes, John said that playing with psychedelics may have opened his mind—and body—to risky behavior. "Some people's minds were not elastic," John said. "They were very rigid and they broke very easily."

John and his friends would attend free concerts in Golden Gate Park. Few of them held jobs. They'd watch bands like Jefferson Airplane and the Grateful Dead. They'd hang around with each other, live together, get some pot, get high, get high on something else, and share food, drugs, sex, and needles. Haight-Ashbury "was not like a vacation place. This was a lifestyle," he said. "Here you are, you're in your twenties, and what are you going to do when you get high? You're going to fuck. Then you're going to do some more drugs. You do some more drugs and somebody's going to get fucked. Bodily fluids are going to get passed."

In 1974, when he was living in the Sunset area near Golden Gate Park, he was feeling ill. He visited a clinic at the University of California, and the doctor gave him a blood test. When the results came back the doctor told John, "There's something going on here. I don't quite understand this. I want you to bring in the people you've been intimate with in the last six months."

The next day John visited two different bars that were his hangouts near the park and Haight-Ashbury. He roamed each bar, stopping at tables and talking with women he had slept with. He also talked with male friends who had been intimate with the same women. He asked them to meet him at a specific time outside the clinic.

The following morning John's friends arrived and traipsed into the clinic. "What the fuck is going on?" the doctor said. He appeared startled, John recalled.

John had brought seventy-two people with him. "It was like a party," he told me.

The doctor knew John had previously been ill with hepatitis A. He said the illness was probably a result of John's earlier infection, but he warned him about too much casual sex. That convinced John to change his lifestyle. "Start using your head ahead of your dick. We don't have to die at forty," John told himself. But it was too late for him to avoid hepatitis C.

# 1968–1974

## SEX

BESIDES CAUTIONING AGAINST promiscuity, health agencies warn that rough sex increases the risk of blood-to-blood contact, which is the only way to catch hepatitis C. Peter was promiscuous, and I had it rough.

I encouraged his promiscuity because of his roughness. I was sexually naive when I met Peter and yearned for more than Kevin's monotonous quickies. But what I got wasn't what I wished for either.

About a week after I met Peter, we rented a sprawling apartment in Flushing, Queens, with several other hippies. As I was unpacking boxes, I carried a stack of linens into the storage room. Right in front of me, Peter and my good friend Teena were rolling around on a sleeping bag. I was still officially married to Kevin and my relationship with Peter was new, so I closed the door and walked out. That evening in our bedroom, Peter said, "I'm a man and I need sex, but I don't care about other women. With you it's different. The universe has given us a special bond."

"Okay," I said. My new partner cuddled against me, even though he seldom liked to cuddle.

That set the sexual parameters for the rest of our relationship. It was the free love era, which applied to fifty percent of the two of us. During our five-and-a-half-year relationship Peter had sex with at least thirty of my friends and probably four or five times as many women I didn't know. He had charisma, and many people, knowing nothing of Peter's personal demons, considered him a guru. Gurus appealed to a lot of hippie women. Often my women friends would tell me about their hijinks with him, as if it

97

were normal. I remember my friend Shirley saying to me, "Peter came over and asked me to give him head. So I did. He said it was okay with you."

Other friends would provide explicit details, and one even asked if Peter was as pushy with me as he had been with her. I shrugged my shoulders. After all, how could I compare our experiences? I was distressed but said nothing to Peter, believing I had implicitly allowed him to fool around when I let the incident with Teena slide.

After the midpoint of our relationship, Peter and I began experimenting with the sacramental use of LSD. We believed the universe had been formed from the eternal dance of the clear light and the void, and we felt we could observe the ballet by ingesting acid. We followed guru Ram Dass, who taught his disciples to "be here now." We studied Zen Buddhism. We searched for the clear light, following Ram Dass's teachings and the Tibetan Book of the Dead. We learned to prepare ourselves for an acid trip, cleaning our apartment, leaving the kids with a babysitter, playing gentle music, and placing bowls of seedless grapes on the table for sweetness and nourishment. We saw LSD as an aid to expanding the mind while clearing the ego.

Eventually, the demons in Peter's past flared up at him. While I searched for the Buddhist version of nirvana, he privately switched to a Hindu god. Visions of Kali infiltrated his psychedelic experience. One evening, after we had each swallowed a tiny translucent square of windowpane acid, Peter declared that I was the many-armed god. He claimed I would destroy the world. He pounced on me, ripped my elephant-print blouse, pulled up my skirt, tore off my underwear, and raped me, brutally, recklessly.

"Stop! I'm not Kali," I shouted. "You're hallucinating!"

He didn't stop. He got rougher.

I struggled to twist away from his grip. "I don't want to do this if you don't think I'm me," I shrieked. "Stop!"

He slammed me into the wall and continued the bruising rape. I watched the controlled, colorful dance of the harmonious energy of the universe slide into a frightening chaos where I was overpowered by a large, venomous man.

I avoided Peter for weeks and tried to think of ways to get myself and my children away from him. But eventually I forgave him. He was good with the kids, and after all, he had been tripping. He had succumbed to a hallucination that wasn't his fault, I believed. I felt we needed to begin anew and suggested we leave Montreal. In the late summer of 1972, we moved to Vancouver.

We started an in-the-basement jewelry manufacturing business. Peter had learned from his father to set cabochon stones in silver and gold mountings, and he was good at it. I was his apprentice and bookkeeper. We wholesaled jewelry throughout British Columbia.

Then he started disappearing an hour here, three hours there. Customers complained he was leaving scratches on metal. Custom orders were going unfilled. The few pieces he made were often cocaine spoons or straws like the one Andrew Loog Oldham described. I received bills for diamonds we had never used in our jewelry and later learned Peter was getting them from wholesalers and selling them at pawnshops to pay for cocaine. I also learned later that he had been shooting the drug into his veins. He had replaced his drive for perfection in his work with an urge for more cocaine. He began to act overly dominant in bed, not raping me but close to it—close to it because I didn't want it, but not quite rape because I said nothing and endured it. After all, I was yet to learn about the coke, he remained gentle with the kids, and I was uncertain of how I could support them alone. He would pummel me night after night and often coaxed me into the bedroom in the daytime too. He would pound at me, not caring about my pleasure, not ever kissing me. I would tuck the kids in for a nap or for bedtime and wind up in bed sooner than I'd wished. I'd close my eyes and Peter would grab me by the hips and pound into me. After a while he would revert to the Kevin position and stay with it for a long, long time. Then he'd just stop. After two or three hours, half asleep, I'd be raw. Raw equals rough in hepatitis terms.

During that time I visited the library and learned that Peter may have been suffering from priapism. It's an often painful condition that causes persistent erections, unrelated to sexual arousal. The Mayo Clinic recommends medical treatment if the erection lasts more than four hours. Oddly, a drug interaction involving an early direct-acting antiviral for hepatitis C, boce-previr, was associated with priapism.[3] The drug was a common treatment for HCV from 2011 through 2013, four decades after my involvement with Peter. But of course, there were no antivi-rals targeting HCV in the '70s. Rather, cocaine would have been a more likely cause of Peter's condition. Chronic use of the drug can deplete norepinephrine from the nerves, leading to priapism. But I didn't know Peter was abusing cocaine until later, when his habit got dangerous.

After a month or so of Peter's mind-numbing coitus style, thoughts of the LSD rape roiled up in me. Although I had forgiven him at the time because he was hallucinating, I kept thinking about his forcefulness that night and how he had physically hurt me. I shied away from his advances and encouraged him to seek other women. He had always fooled around, yet he guarded me as if I were a kitten and all other men were coyotes set to attack. My sex life was disheartening but I was okay with his having sex with other women.

In our large rented townhouse in Vancouver's Kitsilano neigh-borhood, we slept in an extra-wide bedroom. We kept a twin mattress along the far wall, where I would sometimes nap to be away from the sunny window over our bed. One morning, I woke on the larger bed and saw Peter tumbling on that mattress with a sandy-haired woman. I closed my eyes and pretended to go back to sleep. On another occasion, my doctor drove me home after I had a tonsillectomy. I was foggy from painkillers and couldn't find my keys. I stumbled down the block to a friend's house, which was unlocked. I walked in and saw Peter tangled with my friend Marcie on the couch. I walked out and convinced a neighbor to help me climb through my window.

At one point I got a chance for some free love of my own. Our friends James and Anna had been staying in our basement while they searched for an apartment. I went to bed early one night, and Peter and James and Anna stayed up. I awoke in the morning feeling a warm body pressed behind me. Peter was never a cuddler, and I wondered at the change in him. But something about the firm flesh that cupped me felt different. Straight before my eyes, on the spare mattress at the far end of the room, Peter and Anna humped away under a sheet. Anna turned her head and smiled at me, signaling that nothing was wrong. I knew without looking that James was in bed with me. I rolled to face him. I inhaled his scent. He kissed me gently on the lips. I told myself, James is a very nice guy, I like his long, lean body, and I assume Peter wants me to do this. So I did. James was both gentle and passionate. Afterward we hugged, and I saw Peter, still under the sheet with Anna, staring at me.

In the morning, after my daughters had breakfast, the four adults lingered over cups of herbal tea. Peter spouted on and on about harmony and peace. He said we'd all be a family together, forever. He described a wonderful life in the future, including a farm where we'd grow our own food. I left to drop the kids off at another mom's house for a playdate. When I got home James and Anna were gone. Boxes and bags of their belongings were piled on the sidewalk outside the house. Peter raged at me for sleeping with James. He said if he ever saw James again, he'd kill him.

Within a week James and Anna had split up, and I ran into James at a nearby vegetarian restaurant. He sat alone by the Naam's bright front window, eating a veggie burger. I joined him at his table. He said he loved me and wanted to take me and the children away and build a life for us. I liked James a lot, and this could have been my ticket to flee from Peter. But James proposed that he continue working at a sales job and save money for a year before we left. A year was much too long for me, so I said no.

Not long after that I found a note on my door from a cocaine dealer, demanding that Peter pay up. Within an hour, I had thrown together some belongings and moved with my children to my friend Sonya's home, a few blocks away. Until that day, I didn't dodge sex with Peter altogether. Is it possible—although the chances are small—he caught hep from sharing a cocaine needle or from engaging in promiscuous activities and passed it along to me?

## CHAPTER 6

# MILLIONS
# OF VIRIONS

Ⅰ N 1971, WHILE I lay unconscious waiting for a transfusion, the medical system had yet to screen donated
blood for hepatitis C. Scientists hadn't even identified
it as a distinct disease. During the 1960s and early 1970s,
people who needed blood transfusions had a good chance
of getting bad blood.

During that time, Dr. Harvey Alter, of the National
Institutes of Health, was puzzled by high hepatitis infection rates among patients who had received open-heart
surgery. Most of them showed no symptoms of hepatitis,
but their blood tests revealed abnormal liver enzymes. He
later discovered that many of the infected group went on
to develop cirrhosis. Dr. Alter, now a slim older man with
a shiny pate, found that half of the patients who received
at least one unit of blood from a paid blood donor would
contract hepatitis. (He also found a 33 percent hepatitis

infection rate among people who had received any paid donated blood.)

Most paid donors were either in prison or in dire need of cash. A study conducted in California and published in 1966 found ten times as much hepatitis among prison and skid-row blood sellers as among volunteers.

Dr. Alter's research brought up another conundrum. A and B were the only types of hepatitis known at the time. It was impossible to develop hepatitis A through blood transfusions, and Dr. Alter found that only 25 percent of people who had contracted hepatitis through transfusions tested positive for hepatitis B. What was going on? By 1975, Alter and his team began calling the mystery infection "non-A and non-B hepatitis," and many medical people thought it was not a distinct disease but just an odd mix of liver enzymes. It took a decade for researchers to determine that the anomalous illness was a single, separate disease. They named it hepatitis C.

Then, in 1988, Michael Houghton at Chiron Corporation, based in Emeryville, California, managed to clone HCV. The following year the company developed a test that could eliminate the disease from the blood supply. Nonetheless, it took several years before transfusion blood was clear of hep C's viral RNA.

Hepatitis C is an RNA virus, whereas some viruses, such as herpes and chicken pox, are DNA based. Normal DNA (deoxyribonucleic acid) is a stable molecule that safeguards the body's genetic code, whereas RNA (ribonucleic acid) is a less stable code carrier. RNA copies genes and transmits a gene's code to ribosomes, which make proteins within a cell. But it makes many more mistakes (up to a thousand times more) than DNA and does far less error checking. In the midst of the relative RNA free-for-all, hep C virions can alter their surface structure and evade antibodies.

Today, many different tests can count the number of RNA bits in the blood. On April 8, 2014, the day I learned my blood contained antibodies for hepatitis C, Dr. Radev sent me for a polymerase chain reaction (PCR) viral load test, which measures the amount of genetic material in a milliliter of blood. The test uses a polymerase enzyme to copy segments of RNA up to thirty times to gauge the concentration of hep C virions in the blood. When I returned to see Dr. Radev five weeks later and she told me I had hep, she said I had 20,000 bits of viral RNA in each milliliter of my blood. My stomach turned upside down. I felt as if there were armies of grubby little demons scurrying through my system. The examining room seemed to spin haphazardly.

I realized later that, on the one hand, 20,000 was an extremely low load of hepatitis C RNA, but on the other hand, I actually did have millions of viral bits in my blood. A woman of my weight, which dipped to 108 pounds when I was diagnosed, would have about 3,200 milliliters of blood in her body. Although I have always hated math, I hated hep more, and eventually I was curious enough to do this calculation:

20,000 viral load × 3,200 milliliters of blood = 64 million individual hepatitis C viral bits in my body.

It's a good thing I didn't do that equation until long into my treatment. It would have tormented me. Yet 64 million bits of RNA in the big scheme of the body wouldn't matter much—and wouldn't be much matter. Millions of hep C viruses can sit on the head of a pin. About 20 percent of people with hepatitis C have a 6 million viral load per milliliter, not even a full pinhead.

Viruses are teeny, weeny, tiny things. Most are 20 nanometers (0.0000008 of an inch) to 400 nanometers in diameter; the rare, unusually large virus can be about twice that size. The hep C virus is on the small side, between 30 and 75 nanometers across.

In contrast, a red blood cell is 10,000 nanometers in diameter. An ordinary microscope will magnify red blood cells, but even an electron microscope cannot show the hep C virus. It's smaller than a wavelength of violet light (400 nanometers), the shortest wave in the visible spectrum. In fact, nobody really knows what hepatitis C looks like. Electron cryomicroscopy, in which virions are frozen, can show HCV's chemical structure. Graphic artists and scientists come up with images based on the structure.

An image search on Google brings up pictures of the virus that appear almost pretty. Hepatitis C consists of a tiny string of ribonucleic acid enclosed in a viral ball with E proteins sticking out. The pictures usually show perfect spheres with symmetrical projections that spike out like snowflake tines, commonly in the artist's choice of bright rainbow colors. Some of the pictures remind me of Christmas tree ornaments. They remind me of that day when I cut my face with a razor. I didn't cry after the razor cuts, not just because my father yelled at me, but also because the slits had been sleek. I didn't cry when I learned I had hepatitis C. I was dazed, and my world turned upside down and inside out, but like those razor cuts, the disease gave me no physical pain.

Or maybe it did. Maybe my infection caused pain in my arm or stomach, but I was clueless about the source. The initial effects of chronic hepatitis C can be elusive and confusing. People with liver disease may notice itchy skin or feel fatigue, for example, but these feelings are subjective. Hep C can hide in the body for decades. At some point it may produce vague, intermittent, or persistent symptoms, yet most could be seen as symptoms of another illness or even as a figment of the patient's imagination. The imagination can go wild when you're diagnosed with hepatitis C. I'd had some odd physical manifestations during the last few years before my diagnosis. When I finally knew I had hep, I wasn't sure that those physical problems were actually connected with the disease. Then again, once I emerged from the terror that followed diagnosis, my gut said the symptoms were the demon's fault. They may have stemmed from tendinitis, muscle injury, acid reflux, or overwork, but the virus seemed to make them worse.

Between 40 and 75 percent of people who have hepatitis C don't know they have it.[1] Most of them are baby boomers. In the United States, one out of one hundred people has been infected with hep C, and one out of thirty baby boomers is afflicted with the virus.[2] The Mayo Clinic says baby boomers are five times as likely to have hepatitis C as all other adults. Many of them may attribute their symptoms to getting older. The baby boomers are certainly getting older, but those with hep C who don't know it are not getting better.

Dr. Curtis Cooper, the director of the Ottawa Hospital Research Institute and the hospital's Hepatitis Program, sees a lot of hepatitis C patients who have gone without symptoms for decades. He said that after most people are infected, "they don't present to their health care professional saying 'I don't feel well. Test me for something.' If people feel well they don't go see a doctor." Many doctors aren't thinking of hepatitis C, either, he said. "If the patient looks okay or they're dealing with other problems they [doctors] don't think to ask about past risk factors. If it's not thought about, it's not tested for."

That may have been what Dr. Halliman had been thinking—or not thinking. I never complained to her about symptoms except for shoulder pain, which I attributed to an incident in the desert, and sleep problems, which I attributed to the shoulder pain. That's common for people infected with HCV. Most of them die of other causes before the hep rears its head, and many never know of their infection. Sometimes people may have symptoms but fail to recognize them as such. Yet almost everyone I talked with who knew they had hepatitis C confessed to near-obsessive symptom checking once they had been diagnosed. I was no exception. By midsummer 2014 I had fallen into a fanatical symptom hunt. I'd go on the Internet and search for hours for symptoms that might have appeared before my diagnosis and that should have tipped me off. The most frightful was brain fog.

Besides my cooking difficulties, I'd been having trouble teaching classes and found it almost impossible to multitask. I concluded the hep must have affected my brain. Questions about this phenomenon have been drifting through the hepatitis C community for years. Many doctors, researchers, and advocates assert that memory problems, confusion, and irritability caused by hep C seldom occur in people in the early stages of the disease but rather are a symptom of decompensated cirrhosis. But some studies suggest that brains can become foggy well before advanced liver damage sets in. A group of seven researchers in Europe found that 50 percent of hepatitis C patients, regardless of their stage of liver damage, suffer cognitive problems. These include fatigue and difficulties in maintaining attention and recalling information. The study, published in the *World Journal of Gastroenterology,* explains that the body's cytokine proteins direct the immune system to attack HCV. This causes systemic inflammation that can cross the blood–brain barrier. The study suggests that brain fog is a chronic effect of the virus and not a permanent change in the brain.[3]

Researchers have shown not only that treatment can clear the virus but also that it has the potential to clear the fog no matter when it starts. One such study, at Harvard's Beth Israel Deaconess Medical Center, looked at fifteen HCV patients plus seven patients in a control group. None of the patients had cirrhosis. The researchers examined the patients' brain functions using magnetic resonance spectroscopy and gave them multiple tests to evaluate memory, learning, and other cognitive skills. The study, completed in 2011, found that patients who cleared the virus improved their brain functioning but those who failed to clear it did not.

A 2013 study with 150 participants found similar results. Michael R. Kraus et al. tested 150 hep C patients, 90 percent of whom did not have cirrhosis. The tests looked at alertness, divided attention, sustained attention, and working memory. The researchers concluded that hepatitis C affects neuropsychological performance and that the impairment "is potentially reversible after successful virus eradication." They suggested not only that treatment for hep C should be considered in the presence of liver damage but that it should also be considered as a way to unfog the brain.

I dwelled excessively on the brain fog issue, thinking I could endure pain as long as I had a brain. Meanwhile, I learned of some other symptoms of liver disease I may have had:

- Hair becomes sparse under the arms, especially in women. Sometime in the last couple of years preceding my diagnosis, my underarm hair disappeared. Once the virus abated, my armpits again sprouted fine brown filaments. The hair remains thinner than before, which is fine with me.
- Joints may become painful and arthritic. Mine did, but then again, this may have been unrelated to hepatitis C. An MRI showed I had arthritis, tendinitis, tendinosis, and a torn infraspinatus muscle, which is under the shoulder blade.
- Pain can be felt in the liver region. I experienced mild pain, like a bruise, in my right upper abdomen on and off for several months. According to the U.S. Department of Veterans Affairs, hepatitis C can cause anything from a dull ache to severe pain in the liver area. The pain may be intermittent or continual. The department attributes the pain to the stretching of the outer edge of the liver.

The liver pain especially made me worry about how I had treated that vital organ. Alcohol is bad for it, even if you don't have hep. I thought about my foolish bout of drinking on the Yucatán Peninsula. My usual pattern had been to drink a glass or two of wine a few nights a week with dinner. That isn't considered problem drinking, but the margarita madness might have been enough in a small person like me to push a hep-riddled liver into the cirrhotic zone. Because I am a woman, my hepatitis was more likely to be mild than that of a man of the same age. But alcohol can make a woman's liver disease progress more quickly than the liver disease of a man with similar drinking habits.

Liver damage occurs most rapidly when a person contracts hep C after age forty, is a man, and drinks more than

50 grams of alcohol (about two large glasses of wine or three cans of beer) per day. According to the U.S. Department of Veterans Affairs, a man who is infected at age forty-two and drinks a lot can expect a cirrhotic liver in thirteen years. The slowest progression occurs among non-drinking women who contract the disease early. A woman who becomes infected with hep C at age twenty-two (my age when I had a postpartum transfusion) and seldom drinks alcohol has an average wait of forty-two years before the disease turns deadly.

That would mean I'd progress into cirrhosis at age sixty-four, which was exactly my age when I was diagnosed. But the party week in Mexico may have hastened my disease.

Alcohol speeds up the progress of hepatitis C by stimulating the nuclear factor kappa protein, which triggers the virus to replicate. This allows more copies of the virus to swarm through the bloodstream. Alcohol also can poison liver cells and can even lead to alcoholic hepatitis without the help of the virus. In the presence of HCV, the effects of alcohol on the liver are much worse. Alcohol increases inflammation and the rate of fibrosis (liver scarring) that occurs with hep C. It can cause a buildup of iron in body tissues that may induce fibrosis. It creates oxidative stress, an excess of free radicals in the cells accompanied by a shortage of antioxidants. Those are the anticancer, anti–coronary heart disease molecules that health magazines say are good for you. You get antioxidants in foods such as garlic and walnuts, which are on my Good for the Liver List (see the Appendix). Alcohol is at the top of my Bad for the Liver List, followed by two more no-no's: drugs that contain acetaminophen (Tylenol) and prescription drugs with liver warnings.

Everyone I talked with who had hepatitis C said they gave up all of these things immediately and totally when they were diagnosed. They were rightfully scared. Liver disease can linger in the background for years and then suddenly explode because a person has been drinking too much, swallowing liver-damaging drugs, or, in the case of a woman, moving past menopause. In recent years—including the nonstop week of boozing in Mexico—I had done all three. In the two years before my diagnosis, I had tried many painkillers for my shoulder. At least half of them included Tylenol, which in more than normal doses can damage the liver—especially when combined with alcohol. I had also taken Lamisil (terbinafine HCL), which is contra-indicated for persons with liver disease.

About a decade before I learned of my hep C, I came down with the dreaded disease onychomycosis—dreaded by women who want to show off their toenails, that is. My toenails weren't pretty to begin with, but they looked a lot worse with the hard, yellow-brown edges that appear with toenail fungus. The fungus doesn't cause an itch or pain, but it's unsightly. Thinking I was otherwise healthy, I visited Dr. Halliman and asked her to examine my feet.

"I hear there are pills for this," I said as I bared my feet below the examination-room chair. I pointed to my brownish right pinkie toenail and the one next to it, which showed the worst effects of the fungus. I'd be traveling to Florida soon to visit my family. I wanted my feet to look presentable in sandal-land.

Dr. Halliman scribbled the name of the drug on a prescription pad. When I picked up the three-month supply of Lamisil tablets, the druggist gave me a printed sheet warning that Lamisil could harm the liver and should not be taken by anyone who had liver disease. It also said those who take Lamisil should have their liver tested afterward. I remember thinking there was no problem because I was sure my liver was fine.

After three months of Lamisil—which didn't cure my toenails—I returned to Dr. Halliman's office for a checkup. By then I had found my own fungus cure on the Internet: an apple cider vinegar toe-dip twice a day. Dr. Halliman performed the usual checkup procedures, but she didn't suggest that my liver be tested.

I thought nothing of this for years, but soon after I learned I had hep C, I found a letter that Novartis Pharmaceuticals Canada, the manufacturer of Lamisil, had sent to Health Canada about the tablets. It stated, "As of April 2001, based on a Public Health Advisory issued in the U.S., there have been 16 possible Lamisil-associated cases of liver failure, reported worldwide, including 11 deaths and two liver transplantations. In the majority of liver cases reported in association with LAMISIL use, the patients had serious underlying systemic conditions and an uncertain causal relationship with LAMISIL."[4]

Hepatitis C was a serious underlying systemic condition, so I worried about the toenail pills I had used. Had my liver sustained extra damage because I was vain about my feet? Should my doctor have gone beyond face value (or toe value) to make sure my liver was healthy? I had hepatitis C, which no one knew at the time, and it could have been discovered in a toenail medicine follow-up. That might have pushed me toward hep treatment sooner and fended off some of my liver damage.

Just thinking about my liver scared me a lot because I was yet to learn how much damage had occurred. In my last appointment, Dr. Radev had said the specialist would measure my liver scarring. This was commonly done with a biopsy, in which a needle is inserted into the liver. I shuddered at the thought of it, but Dr. Radev had reassured me by saying the gastroenterologist might be able to do a noninvasive test. The result of my genotype test was less than a week away, and at that point I would be getting an appoint-ment with the specialist. I was eager to learn my genotype and even more eager to get rid of the demon, biopsy or not.

Hepatitis C has several genotypes, each with a differ-ent genetic structure. The bits of viral RNA that constitute some hep C genotypes are harder to eradicate than oth-ers. Many of the amazingly effective treatments that were emerging when I was diagnosed could cure one genotype and not another. At that time, for most genotypes, the new inhibitors and antiviral drugs that directly attack HCV had to be combined with the earlier treatment drugs. These were ribavirin, a broad-spectrum antiviral, and interferon, virus-fighting proteins that the body (and also drug com-panies) manufactures. Both could give a patient prolonged, harsh side effects. Interferon is particularly horrific. For many years leading up to 2014, almost everyone treated for hepatitis C had to endure interferon plus ribavirin treatment.

Computer techie Shirley Barger endured it twice. In 1968, at age eighteen, she hopped into her small car in the small town of Hickory, North Carolina, and headed to Cal-ifornia. Shirley's parents had recently died, and she had no home to return to. She pined over her family as she drove. When she arrived in the foggy Sunset district near Golden Gate Park, she was still miserable. She had intended to get a 9-to-5 job, but the music and marijuana scene helped cushion the grief. She picked up work selling an under-ground newspaper on the sidewalks of Haight-Ashbury, where straight-looking tourists gaped at bead-wearing hip-pies like her. Shirley also sold pot.

In 1969 a charismatic man showed her how to inject methamphetamine. She saw the meth as an experiment, and she didn't want to become addicted. Each time she used, she made sure she was clean of the drug before she injected herself again. The dreary comedown told her meth was bad for her, so she stopped using it after her third try.

Unknown to Shirley, the disease had entered her bloodstream. She also caught hepatitis B but fought it off before it became chronic.

Some thirty-five years later, Shirley's hippie times were long gone. She had built a successful career as an assistant administrator of UNIX and Linux systems at the City College of San Francisco, where she enrolled in an HMO. She was feeling tired, more tired than she thought she should be at age fifty-three. She felt a lot of aches and pains. "It just didn't make sense," she said, so she went to see a doctor.

"The doctor decided to test me for everything under the sun except hep C, and for the hell of it I suggested hep C," she said. A friend of hers had contracted the disease, so it came to mind. A nurse practitioner gave her a slip for the test and said, "You wouldn't have that," Shirley recalled.

Shirley told the nurse she didn't think so either.

When Shirley heard the result, she went into "freak-out mode." That was 2003. The Internet wasn't as useful as it is now, so she read book after book about liver disease. Learning about hep and discovering there was a potential cure reassured her somewhat.

She saw a specialist only once before she was treated. "She seemed to be trying to argue with me about whether or not to do treatment," Shirley said. But Shirley insisted that her liver be tested, so she was given a biopsy, which revealed that her fibrosis had reached F2 on the METAVIR scale, a four-level measurement of liver scarring (the F stands for "fibrosis").

Her treatment involved giving herself a weekly injection of Pegasys. It was hard on her, especially because of her finicky job duties. She cut down her working hours but still had trouble. After about a month of interferon and ribavirin, her mind became muddy and she lost half of the college's email system. Luckily, she wasn't fired.

Shirley got sicker the longer she took the treatment. She felt old, decades beyond what an active woman in her mid-fifties should feel. By the time she got to the counter at a grocery store with people darting around her, she practically fell into the shopping cart. She had trouble sleeping and could hardly smell anything, especially food—except for haute cuisine, which would make her stomach spin. As a result, she couldn't enter restaurants and even had trouble walking by them.

Her hair, which was normally wavy, broke off a lot. It became thin and went completely straight until six months after her treatment ended. "It takes several months to a year to get over the effects of the treatment. It's like dedicating two years of your life to it," she said. The dedication didn't pay off.

Twenty-four weeks after the end of the year-long interferon treatment, she had blood drawn for a viral count. The hep had returned. But Shirley was persistent. She wanted to get rid of the disease more than anything and so was willing to endure any hardship.

Next she put herself on a list for clinical studies, and in 2007 a research nurse at the California Pacific Medical Center called her in for a trial. It was for a full interferon treatment, like she had had before, but with a different delivery device. Rather than giving herself shots, an implanted pump in her upper arm would continuously release the drug. Intarcia Therapeutics, which sponsored the trial of Omega DUROS therapy, believed some patients might tolerate interferon better when it entered their body through the device.[5] The DUROS pump had been used in prostate cancer patients to deliver a testosterone antagonist, something that shuts down testosterone, which is known to increase cancer. It had worked well to suppress the male hormone, and cancer patients could tolerate the device for a year at a time. But it was a different story for those with hepatitis C, Shirley said.

The implant in her upper arm looked like a short, tiny pencil under the skin. It could be left in a man for a year at a time to suppress testosterone. Because interferon caused tissue holding the device to break down, however, the device had to be moved several times. At first Shirley was told it would have to be moved every twelve weeks, which would have been four times during her treatment. But she needed surgery to move the little pencil twice as often as that. The doctor would take it out and put a new one in, in the opposite arm. Then six weeks later it would be moved again, into the other arm. Doctors would use a numbing agent during the surgeries, but Shirley was left with cuts that had to heal. "It was pretty weird," she said.

At one point the device got lost. It was supposed to sit just under the skin, but it had migrated deeper. Successively, two doctors tried to get it out but failed. It was moving under their touch and kept sliding away from them. The second doctor called in a plastic surgeon, who pushed a needle into Shirley's arm and listened with a stethoscope for a clunk or a tink, which would mean he was hitting metal. "I had to be extremely still because every time I moved, this thing would migrate a little," Shirley said. "When he hit it I got a little electric shock. He drew the area on my arm and then got it out."

She was agonizingly sick during that treatment. She remembered sitting on the couch at seven-thirty the first night, when all the side effects hit, both physical and emotional. "I was having anxiety attacks and also feeling homicidal. I was feeling homicidal, not suicidal. I wanted to kill." She needed an antidepressant to unwind. She said the treatment had "tons of side effects" but told herself she was so sick that it must be working.

It was still an eleven-month ordeal and the interferon was still combined with ribavirin, but Shirley was optimistic that she would be cured this time. The care while she participated in the trial was much better than in her first treatment. "They pay attention to you," she said. "I thought maybe this would work."

It didn't. Within a month after the forty-eight-week treatment—she was being tested much more often because of the trial—she had relapsed. "The virus was back and pumping away. It's a very tenacious virus," she said.

AFTER HEARING ABOUT interferon's side effects and iffy success rate, some patients refused to take it. Many believed their chances for a cure weren't good enough to try a year-long ordeal of injections, very possible depression, and very probable intense stomach upsets. Pegylated interferon and ribavirin had only a 45 percent success rate in curing genotype 1. Genotypes 2 and 3 did better, with a 75 percent success rate.

The hepatitis C virus mutates quickly and thus often defied interferon's efforts to stomp it out. According to the World Health Organization and many research studies, HCV is an inefficient proofreader. As it copies itself, it makes mistakes, which become variations of the virus. WHO states that rapid mutation is responsible for the chronic form of HCV. As a person's immune system tries to wipe out a particular type of hep RNA, the virus can produce inexact copies. These require different antibodies to attack them. Then the immune system has to create a different defense against the virus, which can change again. After a while, the immune system may give up the fight.

WHO cites six major genotypes of hepatitis C, along with many subtypes of the genotypes. And there are about a hundred strains of these subtypes.

These are the main hepatitis C genotypes and subtypes along with where they are most likely to be found:

1a – North and South America
1b – Europe and Asia
2a – Japan and China
2b – U.S. and Northern Europe
2c – Western and Southern Europe
3a – Australia and South Asia
4a – Egypt
4c – Central Africa
5a – South Africa
6a – Hong Kong, Macau, and Vietnam

TWO WEEKS AFTER blood was drawn to test my genotype, I visited Dr. Radev. She said I had genotype 1b. My virus had probably come from Europe or Asia. Perhaps my blood donor was an immigrant, or maybe the blood had been shipped to Canada. I soon learned I was lucky to have that genotype.

But I didn't feel lucky that day. I still quivered from the shock of diagnosis. Nonetheless, treatment was getting closer. That day Dr. Radev's office confirmed my referral to Dr. Alnoor Ramji, a gastroenterologist. He had been asked to fast-track me because of my waning health insurance. Outside on the sidewalk, I fixed my eyes on the parking lot and took a deep, calming breath. I held it for seven seconds, as I had been instructed in yoga class. Needles, biopsies, and anything else didn't matter anymore. I would do whatever the specialist said to get rid of my awful disease.

On May 28, 2014, the day after I learned my genotype, I called Dr. Ramji's office. His assistant answered. She said my appointment would be on August 25. Nadia's voice was soothing, but her answer was not. My jitters returned full force. That was three months away! Three months of demon micro-bugs constructing dirty, scraggly litter piles in my liver and roping them together to clutter the once spotless organ with grimy debris.

I chatted with Nadia for a while, telling her the story of my transfusion and learning that she was devoted to her job and the patients. She said that Dr. Ramji was a very nice man and that the clinic would take good care of me. I felt like I had made a friend but hadn't made much progress toward a cure. I had no idea of how much liver damage I was facing, but I'd be having an ultrasound of my liver soon. That would tell me something, I hoped.

Two days later I arrived at St. Mary's Hospital (now called the Sechelt Hospital) for an ultrasound. A liver ultrasound is an easy, comfortable procedure. As a friendly woman in a green smock rolled a gel-coated transducer on the skin over my liver, I relaxed. She also scanned my gallbladder, a pear-shaped organ attached to the liver that breaks down fat. Hepatitis C can inflame the gallbladder, causing pain when a person eats fatty foods.

Before I knew it, she was done. "Your doctor will have the results in a week or so," she said.

The thirty-minute drive home from the hospital took me through the town of Sechelt and along the Sunshine

Coast Highway, past long expanses of forest that overhang the road, past rocky beaches, past the commercial area of Upper Gibsons, and down a long hill toward the ferry terminal; my home is just past the terminal. When I arrived I was no longer calm. I had been doing too much thinking. A week seemed like a long, long time. The specialist's appointment, more than thirteen weeks away, seemed an impossible wait. A week later, I called Nadia, and she put me on the cancellation list. I waited.

# DESERTION

BARELY A WEEK after I returned to New York City from the Virgin Islands, my parents' offer to buy me a restaurant disintegrated. They were angry that I had left my husband and had shacked up with a man who was evading the Vietnam War. Added to that, Peter, my daughter, and I were living with several hippie friends, including another mom and child, in a large Manhattan apartment. I got a job as a secretary for a holding company in the Park Avenue business district and shared babysitting with the other mom, and little Della always had little Lenore to romp with. Life, to me, was good. My parents called again and again, demanding that I return home. I refused again and again.

One evening my youngest sister called.

"What do you mean, we're getting busted?" I asked Irene.

"Our father is on the way there with his cop friends," she said.

"What do you mean? He said he was buying me a restaurant."

"I don't think so," Irene said. She lived with my parents and eavesdropped when she could.

Irene's warning began to make sense. The restaurant had been a ruse to lure me to New York. My adrenalin level soared. I hung up the phone. "Get up! Get up! Cops are coming!" I shouted.

"The cops?" Peter asked, stumbling out of the bathroom where he had been dealing with a bout of nausea.

"Yes! My dad's bringing them."

Peter's yellowish face turned white. The rest of us could protect ourselves by getting rid of the weed, but that wouldn't keep an army deserter out of the brig. Despite his possible attack of island-spawned hepatitis, Peter raced like a wildebeest out of the apartment.

Brendan and Susye pulled up the sofa cushions. They peered under the edges of the hand-knotted rug that covered part of the living room.

I checked on the little ones. Della hugged a stuffed doggy doll. Lenore hugged a blanket. They were oblivious to the frenzy in the apartment. I closed their door quietly and let them sleep, then beelined to the coffee table, grabbed a nickel bag of marijuana ($5 worth, about a quarter of an ounce), and replaced it with a burning stick of incense.

Brendan, Susye, and Ryan rummaged through the kitchen. They checked every container of beans and rice—we were into beans and rice—and bag of produce, in case someone had inadvertently hidden something in a food container. They checked all the spice jars, in case the oregano that looked like pot was really pot. Ryan yanked a couple of green-filled baggies from a cupboard. I joined him in the bathroom with the little manila nickel bag. The weed swirled down the toilet. We ripped the baggies and the envelope into shards and flushed them away too.

There was pounding at the door. The bearded man who had rented us the suite opened it, keys jangling from his hand. He stepped aside, and three burly cops stormed in with my dad behind them. My friends stood together at the far end of the hall, blocking the living room.

It was my father who had brought the cops, so I felt it was my responsibility to speak. "You can't come in here," I said.

"Yes, we can. Get out of our way," said a big huff of a cop with a blond brush cut and huge ears sticking out. He shoved me to the side and stomped down the hall past my friends. The other two cops followed.

"Why are you doing this?" I asked as my dad limped past me, avoiding my eyes.

His grimace looked as if it had been pasted onto his face. His mouth stayed clamped.

Big Ears stomped around the living room. He lifted the sofa cushions and moved toward the center of the room. My dad followed and helped him pull up the rug. Another cop yanked down from the ceiling the mandala sheets we used as room dividers, as well as two strings of homemade lampshades. The cop and my dad trampled the lampshades. They unzipped everyone's bags and tossed clothing all over the floor.

The cop with the acned face was tearing up the kitchen. It had a double-size opening into the living room, so I could see what was going on. He pulled a hefty bag from a cupboard. Whole-wheat flour whooshed over the kitchen floor and dusted into the living room. Acne Face lumbered toward a bedroom, leaving a trail of brownish white footprints. He was about to open the door to where the kids were sleeping.

"Where's your warrant?" I asked. "You shouldn't be here without a warrant."

"We don't need one, sister," Big Ears said.

"I know you need one. I'm calling my lawyer." I didn't have one, but I grabbed the phone and started dialing. All three cops turned their eyes to my father and headed toward the exit.

"Keep looking! You can't leave," he told them.

"Sorry, Joe. We'd better go," Big Ears said.

My dad scowled and followed his cop friends out the door. Their visit should have been a warning sign. My big mistake was to stay in the apartment.

Two days later, I had just fed the babies and was getting dressed for work. There was a knock at the door, and I foolishly opened it. One of those cops shoved a subpoena into my hand. My parents were taking me to court to gain custody of my daughter.

I skipped work and cried all day. As I huddled on the sofa gasping, Teena hugged me and stroked my hair. Peter walked in circles, ranting. Harry jumped out of his usual malaise and got on the phone with his brother. He asked Tim to be our pro bono lawyer.

Soon Peter and I sat across from Tim at a staid law office in midtown Manhattan. He passed us a list of about twenty allegations.

My parents' statement of claim said I was living an immoral life and did not have enough clothes for my child. It said I used drugs and associated with drug users. It alleged there were orgies in my apartment. Until I read the legal statement and checked a dictionary, I didn't know what an orgy was. As for the clothes, it was true there weren't enough of them. I had just arrived in New York from the Caribbean. I had bought only a skirt and a dress for my new job and was planning to splurge on children's wear once the first paycheck came in. Until then, most of my daughter's clothes, like mine, were T-shirts and shorts.

"Did your parents observe any of this?" Tim asked.

"Not at all."

"Their suggestions of drugs and immoral behavior are vague and unprovable," he said.

That took care of most of the list. I began to relax. Tim had a gentle manner. He looked a lot like his brother Harry but was clean cut. He opened a thick brown book to a bookmarked page. "There's a law in New York that says if the parents can't afford clothing, the grandparents are obligated to buy it. They can't blame the clothing problem on you. Once both of you testify, the judge will dismiss the case."

Peter glanced sideways at me. He couldn't testify because he was AWOL, he told the lawyer.

"Don't worry," Tim said. But I worried.

About a week later Kevin, my estranged husband, called. He said my father had visited him. He had asked Kevin to testify that I was a bad mother, and he had dangled a bunch of fifty-dollar bills in front of him. Kevin and I had been distant since our breakup, but he had told my dad I was a good mother. He refused the bribe.

Then my friend Diane Duffy visited my apartment. She said my father had called and offered her $800 to testify against me. My stomach sank. What was next? That was big money in those days, equal to about six weeks of my earnings in a secretarial job. Diane had said no. She moved from friend to BFF instantaneously.

The court date arrived and I, but not Peter, walked into the courthouse. I sat on a wooden bench in a corner of a wood-paneled waiting room. My parents showed up with their lawyer, a spiffy older man with a ten-inch-thick briefcase.

Tim arrived. "Don't worry. It's in the bag," he said as we entered the courtroom. The clerk read out procedural matters. The white-haired judge called my lawyer and my parents' lawyer to the podium. They talked quietly. Then the judge rapped his gavel and called a recess.

Back in the waiting room I asked Tim what the talk was all about. "They want to move the proceedings to the end of the day."

That didn't make sense. My parents were staring at me across the room. They must have felt as uncomfortable as I did and would probably want to get this over with quickly. I left to go to the washroom. When I reentered the hallway outside the waiting room, my dad leaned against a wall and I had to pass close to him. As I strode along trying not to see him, tears trickled from his eyes. "You're too young to make these decisions by yourself. I have to do this," he said and turned away.

I waited and waited and waited, staring at the door of the courtroom, sitting right across the twenty-foot room from my parents. Finally, the court clerk called my case. Inside the courtroom the judge banged his gavel and said, "It's late in the day. We're all getting tired and need to eat dinner." He said the case would adjourn until September, and meanwhile my parents would have temporary custody of my daughter.

My mouth hung open. September was four months off. Della would be two at the end of that month. Four months would be a long, long time in her very short life. That would be a long time in my life as well—far, far worse than my unnerving wait for a specialist before my treatment for hep was to be.

My parents took nineteen-month-old Della to their sprawling new home in an upscale area of Flushing, Queens. I was allowed to visit on weekends. When the visiting hour ended, Della would wrap her small arms around my legs and cry. When I got home, I would cry as well. Tears would pool on my pillow as I tried to sleep. I would wake at dawn, sobbing into the wetness, realizing my baby wasn't there. After a few weeks I called a truce with my parents. Peter, Della, and I moved in with them. I took the bus and subway to work in Manhattan each day. Peter planned to surrender to the army by feigning mental illness, the one ailment that might excuse an AWOL.

One bright morning he walked into the emergency room of an army hospital, took a seat in the waiting room, and munched down a square of blotter paper. It contained at least a dozen hits of LSD. Within twenty minutes Peter's pupils dilated to dime-size. He grinned like a circus clown and stomped about the room, spreading and collapsing his arms as if he were trying to collect things that were floating in the air. A team of hospital aides grabbed him and pushed him onto a stretcher. Peter howled and struggled to get off, so they strapped him down. Someone must have called his mother. She arrived hollering at the doctors, demanding they be easy on her son. I knew what was happening and quietly looked on.

The psychiatrists believed Peter was insane, or they believed that taking LSD automatically made people insane. They transferred him to an army psychiatric unit in Pennsylvania, where he was forced to take Thorazine, a strong antipsychotic. Each week-end I would drive to visit him at the hospital. My eyes would water and sting as I drove past the billowing smokestacks of New Jersey's industrial area. My eyes would tear even more as I viewed Peter's fellow patients in the mental ward. Most of them were just out of Vietnam, suffering invisibly from what today is called posttraumatic stress disorder and visibly from bodily losses. At least a third of the dozens of young men I saw in the ward were missing an arm or two, a foot or two, a leg or two, or a combination of parts. I became friends with a man who seemed barely old enough to have enlisted. His hand and leg had been blown off by a mine. I remember him saying it was a good thing the explosion hit his left side and not his right.

"I'm right-handed, hey? I can do a lot of things," he said from his wheelchair as he sipped a Coke with his right hand. I felt that the world had gone crazy, letting the Vietnam War continue to rage. Meanwhile, Peter was so drugged he could barely mumble.

After four or five weeks Peter was discharged from the hospital but not from the army. He would have a short leave and then be sent to Vietnam.

Our friend Ryan had sent some photos from Arizona. One showed a house with gray wood paneling and a wide patio where a bunch of hippies gathered. A long-haired man was playing a guitar, and it appeared as if the rest of them were singing. Another photo showed Ryan dipping a bare foot into a gurgling stream. Leafy green plants burst up near the water.

"How about it?" Peter asked.

"Sure. When do we go?"

"As soon as we can."

"How about tomorrow?"

I had been working full-time at the holding company and had saved up enough to buy plane tickets. Of course we couldn't tell my parents Peter was again deserting.

When they were out for the evening playing bridge, Peter and
I packed two huge duffel bags, a baby's supply bag, and a knap-
sack. Della now had plenty of winter clothes and summer clothes
too. I threw them in a pile on the thick green rug in my bedroom.
Almost everything in my parents' home was green. It was June,
and New York was getting hotter.

"Maybe it's cool in Arizona?" I joked.

"No, but throw in the winter stuff anyway," Peter suggested.
"You never know."

Little did I know that winter clothing would come in handy,
and that soon I'd witness the scariest scene of my life. It would
take place in the desert. Could the demon have ambushed me
there?

CHAPTER 7

# THE TINY
# JACKHAMMER

I FACED THE COMPUTER screen in my basement office. Outside the window, two tall cedar trees formed parallel lines toward the sky. They had been sheared of all branches up to thirty feet in order to reveal the ocean view. Clouds settled over the water, a quiet drizzle fell, and a storm blew through my mind. The demon was thundering through my liver, and my appointment with the hepatologist was two months away. I scoured the Internet, trying to find solace. Skipping from one web page to another, I thought I found good news: "The majority of people with chronic Hepatitis C will never develop a major complication related to this disease."

Reading on, I realized that the statement seemed to apply only to those who had had hep for up to twenty years. The writer, Nicole Cutler, stated, "If undetected, ignored or untreated, Hepatitis C is more likely to develop into cirrhosis or liver cancer."

A case in point: Jim Banta, the San Francisco construction worker who fell from the scaffolding at an elevator shed, learned that he had contracted hepatitis C and on the same day discovered that his liver had advanced to end-stage disease. "That's pretty crazy," he said on the phone to me. About a month after his fall, which broke two ribs, he spent ten days in the hospital, wracked with worry about his diagnosis. End-stage liver disease means what it implies. Jim was at the beginning of the end of his liver's ability to function. The body can't live without a liver, so the only recourse is a transplant.

For the next nine years Jim was never well enough to get a transplant. He was never well enough to endure hep C treatment, either. The standard treatment at the time was interferon, which was likely to make Jim's difficult symptoms much worse. His symptoms from liver failure would spike, level off, and then progressively increase. He was often sick to his stomach, and his thoughts would become blurry. His blood contained too much ammonia, which is produced when the body digests proteins. With a damaged liver, excess ammonia can accumulate. The result is encephalopathy, or overall brain dysfunction, which affects memory, muscle control, and other brain functions. A normal or even fibrotic liver would get rid of ammonia, but Jim's cirrhotic, decompensated liver could not. In 2009 Jim passed out at home, and his wife called an ambulance. He had fallen into a coma.

He was rushed to San Francisco General Hospital, where a shunt was placed through his liver, allowing blood traveling from the intestines to the heart to bypass the tangle of cirrhosis. The procedure worked for Jim. After several days in the coma, he woke up. The hospital stabilized him and transferred him to the UCSF (University of

California–San Francisco) Medical Center Hospital, one of America's leading transplant hospitals. After five and a half weeks at the hospital, he had lost seventy pounds, but he had also learned he would get a liver. Because he still had hep C, he agreed to take a lower-quality liver and so was able to get one much faster than most other people on the transplant list.

"If I had gotten a pristine liver, I would have infected it with my hep C," Jim said. "I said, 'I'll take a liver with hep B. I'll take a liver with hep C. It doesn't matter because I'll infect it anyway.' That broadened my horizons for what was available to me and actually saved my life because I didn't have the time to wait."

The donor had been a twenty-two-year-old woman with hepatitis C whose liver damage was much less extensive than his. The transplant tacked years onto his life. Jim went through three transplants before he was treated with interferon and ribavirin.

From 2012 through 2013 Jim endured more than a year of the dreaded treatment. He was anemic for eight months during the regimen and needed a blood transfusion. "But I always knew that at the end I would be done, whereas the nine years I spent waiting for a liver transplant and getting sicker and sicker and sicker... that was endless and at times almost hopeless," he said. "I had survived a liver transplant, so I wasn't going to let sixty weeks of treatment put me down."

Jim was braver than I. Thinking that I might need a transplant, I was terrified. But I had never been one to get depressed, except perhaps in the previous few years or so when hep C had stepped up its attack. I had lost so much weight it was impossible to hold up a pair of size 2 pants without a belt. (I had been a size 6 previously.) I couldn't sleep more than two hours at night without taking zopi-clone. Complications at work, which I had previously seen as a challenge, had come to seem insurmountable. My dry eyes had become drier. The skin on my legs itched. I could no longer multitask.

The good news was that if I took on only one occupa-tion at a time, I could concentrate as well as ever. The good news was that my favorite task was writing, and research was part of writing. I continued to plow through the Inter-net looking for hope. And hope was there. It came in the form of reports about new direct-acting antivirals that were promising to revolutionize hepatitis C treatment. That news pushed my hand toward the phone. I called Nadia. We chatted about the weather. We said we hoped the skies would clear.

"Am I still on the cancellation list?" I asked.

"Yes, of course. I'll call you as soon as anything comes up."

"Where am I on the list?"

"Oh, let me see," she said. "Oh, yes, it's the Canada Day long weekend, and we've had a few changes. There's an appointment now open for July 10. Can you make it?"

"Sure I can." It was the best news I had heard in a freaked-out month.

So there I was at 10:45 a.m. on July 10, 2014, in the wait-ing room at the Pacific Gastroenterology Associates clinic in downtown Vancouver. I would be seeing Dr. Alnoor Ramji soon. Eight other patients were settled on pink-cushioned chairs that lined three walls of the rectangular room. Most of the patients were my age or older. A frail, stubble-chinned man glanced at me and then returned his gaze to a magazine. I checked email on my phone. I felt jittery. Everyone else seemed to be comfortable as they waited for their names to be called. I guessed I was the only newbie there.

After a few minutes a petite woman wearing a tunic top and black leggings, her black hair pouring down her back, introduced herself as Maria Ancheta-Schmidt, clinical research manager of the GI Research Institute. She led me into the treatment lounge, and for the rest of the year she would guide me toward sustained virologic response (SVR). SVR means a cure.

In the lounge, Maria settled next to me on one of several puffy brown leather armchairs. Beside the armchairs stood head-high stainless steel poles with hooks projecting from the top for hanging intravenous drip bags. I would not need to use one, but I didn't know that at first. Thankfully, Maria said all the right things to reassure me. She said my decades of hidden hepatitis were not unusual. I had an excellent chance of being cured, she said. I learned right away that among Maria's many endearing qualities is optimism, which she slathers with gentle words upon her patients.

Maria manages research organized by pharmaceutical companies that are testing gastrointestinal therapies. She works with doctors involved in research, including my specialist, Dr. Alnoor Ramji, who heads a three-doctor hepatology team.

Maria said her job at the institute, helping hep C patients, has been great, "but I'm working myself out of a job. We're getting an almost 100 percent cure rate, and the treatment's getting easier—one pill a day, less side effects, you're not monitoring labs as much or adjusting any doses. It's getting easier all the time."

That made me more optimistic than anything.

As the liver goes from healthy to fibrotic to cirrhotic, it hardens. The hep C virus invades liver cells, turning them into HCV reproduction factories. Meanwhile, the virus inflames and destroys those cells. Scar tissue forms. The liver's spongy jellyfish texture gradually becomes a hardened network of scars.

In the earliest stage of fibrosis, the scars are isolated and the liver functions as usual. As the scarring proceeds, more and more of the liver is affected. The scars begin to branch, connect, and group. Septa, which are bands of fibrous scar tissue, form. When the damage moves to cirrhosis, regenerative nodules—scar bands that surround clusters of liver tissue—appear. The liver eventually loses its ability to produce proteins, regulate essential chemicals, and clean the blood of toxins. Only a successful liver transplant will restore those functions.

In the past, liver scarring was assessed through a biopsy or a Fibrosure test. A biopsy involves inserting a needle into the liver to remove a tissue sample. Pathologists will look through the sample with a microscope to determine the amount of scarring. Fibrosure, patented by Laboratory Corporation of America, is a blood test that measures bilirubin and other parts of blood serum that change with liver disease. The results are entered into an equation that factors in the patient's gender and age. The test shows levels of liver damage that correspond to the four stages on the METAVIR scale, from undamaged through cirrhosis. Biopsies had been the more common test and had been required by many health insurers.

After my diagnosis, I worked my way through my fear of getting blood drawn with a hypodermic needle, but the thought of a liver biopsy was far worse. As far as I knew, I might need one. I feared that the needle would be large and that I would feel it as it probed my damaged organ. About half of patients feel pain after a biopsy. Worst of all, I would be awake during the procedure and would have to think about what was being done. Dr. Radev had said my specialist might use an easier method to assess my liver, but I wasn't sure of that. Maria relieved my fears right away, telling me, "You're going for a thump test."

She led me past the reception area to a six-foot-by-eight-foot windowless room that had space for only a small examining table, a stool for a nurse-technician, and a computer console with a narrow vertical screen and a little tool attached to its side. A nurse-technician with fiery red hair wearing a purple T-shirt and flowered skirt came in holding the FibroScan tool. It was the size and shape of a toilet-paper tube, with a small nib at the top. A cord attached it to the computer stand.

She asked me to pull up my shirt to the bottom of my bra and rubbed water-based ultrasound gel below my rib cage on my right. She held the little rod against the spot. I felt a slight thump. There was another thump and another. It reminded me of a tiny jackhammer. But rather than ear-pounding bangs, the FibroScan let out just a faint purr. After ten thumps, the nurse looked at a readout on the computer screen.

As the technician thumps .your liver—usually in the largest of the liver's two lobes—the FibroScan computer determines the organ's median stiffness. Then an algorithm compares this with a set of scores. A FibroScan score, which ranges from zero to 75, indicates whether you have stage 1, 2, or 3 fibrosis or stage 4, cirrhosis. With cirrhosis, regression is less likely and symptoms are more likely to set in. As I watched the nurse watching the FibroScan screen,

I was my optimistic self. I expected to learn that I was at stage 1 or, at the most, stage 2.

A segmented vertical bar appeared on the screen. I had no idea how to interpret the lines, but the technician said matter-of-factly, "You're at level 3."

It took a moment for her words to sink in. I stared at the screen and mumbled, hardly moving my lips, "Okay."

Within seconds I was anything but okay. As my mind plodded through the stage 3 miasma, I was led to Dr. Alnoor Ramji's office. He was standing behind a polished wood desk. He lowered his eyes, as if he were bashful, and then gave me a warm, concerned smile. He held out his hand and asked how I was. In my experience, almost all doctors I've visited for health matters first ask, "How are you?" Maybe they are just defaulting to the customary conversational opening. But maybe they actually want to know if the patient is feeling physically well or if their stomach is aching, if their vision is blurry, or if their foot throbs from stepping on a nail. But I answered the way I assumed most people answer.

"Fine," I said. But I wasn't fine. I imagined those icky, teeny demons having a party in my liver. I pictured them rollicking on bridges of scar tissue and flitting from bridge to bridge. As I shook the doctor's hand and took a seat in front of his desk, the hurt I had felt from Ellen and others who seemed to lack empathy rolled away, at least temporarily. I sensed that Dr. Ramji had great compassion for his patients. I knew I was finally in the good hands of the good doctor whose hand I had shaken.

I also had a sense of déjà vu. It seemed almost as if I had been in this doctor's office before, going through the same introduction. I'm certain that wasn't so, but it was a big day for me, the biggest in my travails with hepatitis C. Learning the extent of my liver damage had been disheartening, but it was a necessary step on the way to breaking up the virus fest. I believed Dr. Ramji would make me get better.

Dr. Ramji told me that after he had completed degrees in pharmacy and medicine, he had studied hepatology, which he found intellectually stimulating. He also realized he could help a lot of people with cirrhosis become well. In addition to the liver's many functions, he said, "It's one of those organs that is somewhat forgiving." If you can halt whatever process is damaging the liver, the organ often begins to heal itself, he explained. "The ability to do that for anything in this world is incredible."

Many studies have verified the starfish-like regenerative ability of the liver. It is the only human organ that can rebuild itself. People can lose up to 75 percent of their liver and have it grow back to a normal size. When a liver is whole but is scarred internally, it can repair the damage. Hepatologists call this *regression*. Researchers from the Institute of Cellular Medicine at Newcastle University in England pored over the most current studies to determine whether liver regression is a fact or just a function of inaccurate liver testing. They found increasing evidence of fibrosis regression and liver regeneration in people who had fibrosis and had been cured of hepatitis C. That day in Dr. Ramji's office, I was hoping for something incredible like that. The doctor asked me about my symptoms, and, ever the optimist, I said I had none.

"Have you lost any weight?" he asked.

I had. I was skinny as a twig compared with my normal weight, which had melted off the year before. "I lost maybe ten pounds last year," I said.

He frowned in concern.

"But I was exercising a lot more than usual," I said. Later, when I thought back to the months when I had lost all the weight, I realized I actually may have been exercising *less* than usual.

Dr. Ramji asked a string of questions, including how much alcohol I drank. I said I drank one or two glasses of wine at dinner some nights, but I forgot to mention the copious amounts I had drunk in Mexico.

He assured me that if my hepatitis were cured, my liver could repair itself. There was no guarantee it would regenerate, but there was an excellent chance of a cure for my hepatitis C, especially with the newest antiviral drugs. He gave me three choices of treatment drugs:

1. 12 weeks of simeprevir plus sofosbuvir
2. 12 weeks of sofosbuvir plus interferon
3. 48 weeks of interferon plus ribavirin

Dr. Ramji said he would prefer that I take number 1, the non-interferon treatment. It had been approved by Health Canada the week before and had done exceptionally well in recent clinical trials for my genotype. The second option would be good too, he said. Number 3, the much longer treatment with interferon and ribavirin, was likely to produce the worst side effects and the least chance of success. However, the newer drugs were expensive, and not many health plans would pay for them. I said I had great health insurance but had already given notice that I was leaving my job, so my coverage would vanish soon. Given that I was stage 3 on the METAVIR scale and at the end stage of my health plan, he assured me, whatever treatment I chose would start quickly.

"I've heard," I said, "that 96 percent of people get cured with the direct-acting antivirals."

They see such percentages in clinical trials, Dr. Ramji said, but I shouldn't expect that kind of result.

Later I talked with other researchers, and they all agreed. Patients in clinical trials have their enzymes, viral load, and vital signs tested more than regular patients in order to provide essential information to make sure the new medicines are safe. The test group receives intense guidance from the research team, including frequent encouragement and support throughout the treatment and afterward. In addition, drug trials include only certain types of patients. For a hepatitis C drug, for example, a trial might include only people who have never been treated for hep C and have scored between 2 and 3 on the METAVIR scale. Another trial might look for only women over fifty or men with genotype 3 who have been infected for ten to twenty years. With all of the factors so well controlled, clinical trials are likely to yield a larger percentage of cures than individual treatments. Ads for hep C antivirals tend to cite the trial results. That increases both demand for the drugs and patients' expectations of a cure.

"So what chance would I have of being cured with the new drugs?" I asked Dr. Ramji.

"Think of it as 80 to 90 percent."

"Eighty-five?"

"About eighty-five," he said.

That sounded better than eighty, and it would be a far greater source of hope than the third option. As I walked past the reception counter to return to the GI Institute, I felt stunned and uncertain. I was glad I'd been fast-tracked but scared that I still might have to settle for option 3. I had heard a lot about interferon, but nothing I knew about it was good.

Despite its debilitating side effects, however, interferon was a lifesaver for many people with hepatitis C. Unfortunately, only about half of those who took the drug for hepatitis C were cured. Some patients, like IT administrator Shirley Barger, underwent many months of interferon treatment, were told their HCV had disappeared, and learned a few months later that it was back. Many other people couldn't endure interferon's side effects and quit treatment early.

Others who stopped treatment, like sociology professor Ben Handley, were able to kick the disease even after quitting interferon early. Ben had given up seven months into a one-year treatment. He was tested every month after that, and after a year his viral load came back negative. He stopped the treatment in April 2009 and went back to work two months later. Work at first was an ordeal, because it took six months to get over the ill effects of interferon. Ben said his liver still contains huge amounts of triglycerides—fatty lipids that can lead to pancreatitis—but this problem is being treated with drugs. There's not as much scarring in his liver, he said. Ben's spouse, Dennis, a robust guy with a shock of blond hair pushed to the side of his forehead, continued to look healthy but would need to get treated for hep one day.

The problems with interferon, which cured around half of patients, spurred research into better drugs. That led to today's antivirals, which can cure almost everybody who has hepatitis C. A combination of interferon, ribavirin, and two protease inhibitors introduced in 2011 upped the cure rate to between 66 and 79 percent.[1] By 2017, close to 100 percent cure rates were possible with direct-acting antivirals for some genotypes and patient groups.

Through late 2014 and early 2015, hepatitis treatment shifted toward a new, one-pill-a-day treatment, free of interferon. I was treated earlier, and the medical profession had yet to abandon that treatment. Interferon had been on my list of potential treatments, but it was there for one reason only. It was—relatively speaking—cheap.

When Dr. Ramji said the new, direct-acting antivirals were very expensive, I thought about some acid-reflux pills I had taken a few years before. The pink esomeprazole tablets allowed me to drink lemonade and eat cashew nuts without getting stomach pains. Sixty days of the anti-acid-reflux drug had cost $130, which I had felt was exorbitant for a small container of pills. It turned out that one esomeprazole tablet cost about one-tenth of a percent of the cost of a day's worth of pharmaceuticals I would swallow to get rid of hepatitis C.

Back in the treatment lounge, I settled into one of the leather chairs and listened to Maria's matter-of-fact explanation of the hep C drugs Dr. Ramji had proposed. His number one choice, simeprevir and sofosbuvir (Dr. Ramji and Maria insisted on using the generic drug names rather than the publicized brand names, Galexos and Sovaldi), would doubtlessly be the easiest on my body. Both simeprevir and sofosbuvir are direct-acting antivirals, which means they directly target HCV rather than just bolster the immune system, like interferon does. Both simeprevir and sofosbuvir keep hep C virions (individual viral particles) from replicating. If the virions die faster than they reproduce, eventually all of them will die and the demon will vanish. But the top-tier drugs were outrageously expensive. Here are the details as they stood at the time:

- Sofosbuvir (brand name Sovaldi) bonds with the virus and blocks the function of the NS5B polymerase, a

protein the hep C virus uses to replicate itself. Sovaldi's main side effects are allergic reactions, depression,
shortness of breath, weakness, and pale skin. The drug
was selling at $1,000 a pill in the U.S., for a total of
$84,000 for a twelve-week treatment. As a Canadian
I was lucky, if you could call my situation lucky. The
Canadian government negotiates with drug companies
and had lowered the cost for patients to about $68,000.
Gilead Sciences makes Sovaldi.

- Simeprevir, a protease inhibitor, is called Olysio in the
  U.S. and Galexos in Canada. Simeprevir blocks an HCV
  protein, NS3/4A serine protease, which is crucial in
  viral replication. The main side effects of simeprevir are
  allergic reaction, shortness of breath, skin redness, skin
  irritation, mouth sores, and eye irritation. Developed by
  the Belgium-based Janssen Pharmaceuticals, simeprevir
  cost $66,000 in the U.S., $47,000 in Canada, for a
  twelve-week treatment.

The total cost of the two drugs would be about $115,000.
Add to that the pharmacy's dispensing fee, and I could
expect to pay about $120,000 for treatment. Maria advised
that I talk with the people in charge of my medical plan right
away to see if it would pay for the sofosbuvir-simeprevir
drug combination.

"But the side effects sound harsh," I said.

Don't worry, she said, most of the effects showed up in
trials that included interferon. She said that if I were to
take the two drugs on their own, side effects from both of
the direct-acting antivirals were likely to be minimal. She
emphasized again that the worst problem could be the cost.

The second choice Dr. Ramji had offered was sofosbuvir plus interferon. Maria assured me this option would be

much easier than interferon alone. Interferon's side effects usually take a few weeks to emerge. The sofosbuvir would reduce the forty-eight-week interferon treatment time (for genotype 1b) to twelve weeks. I would be practically finished with treatment before heavy side effects kicked in, Maria said. Twelve weeks of interferon would cost about $6,000, but I'd also have to pay for sofosbuvir. That was still in the financial stratosphere for me. However, it seemed more likely that an insurance company would cover the sofosbuvir-plus-interferon combination than the non-interferon first choice. Health Canada had just approved the two-drug antiviral combination, but the province considered it an "off-label treatment." Canadian doctors may prescribe off-label prescriptions, but insurance companies seldom allow them.

Treatment number three was interferon with ribavirin. Despite potential awful side effects, it was still considered the standard treatment, and most health plans would pay for it. Pegylated interferon plus ribavirin would cost only $420 a week in Canada, about double that in the U.S., but with my hard-to-kill genotype I'd have to endure forty-eight weeks. Although $20,000 was a pittance compared with the other options, interferon had sunk to the deep, grungy bottom of my wishing well.

I had already signed off on the end of my employment, yet I wanted the most effective and easiest treatment. That meant the most costly drugs. Paying for them would ravage my retirement fund. My hope lay in my insurance company and in the drug companies' patient support programs. Maria advised me to talk with people at my health care plan and at the patient support programs for both Sovaldi (sofosbuvir) and Galexos (simeprevir), and to get another blood test, since she would need to know my baseline viral load before I began treatment. I would have to have another PCR viral load test done each week during the regimen. But the blood tests would be easy compared with negotiating the payment maze.

I spent the next several days struggling to come up with money to pay for the prescription and the next several nights tossing and barely sleeping. The demon tormented me and shoved me into my past. I told myself the blood transfusion I had received after childbirth was the likely source of the hep. But I had been a happy new mother. Being diagnosed with hepatitis C isn't a happy event, so my gut questioned that explanation. I thought through my sexual stupidity with Peter. I should never have left New York with him and gone with him into the desert.

**Early July 1969**

# CANYON

AS PETER AND I packed for the flight to Arizona, I called the holding company where I worked. "My aunt's very sick. I have to move to Arizona immediately," I told my boss. "Would you please send my final paycheck to the Western Union office in Kingman?" Western Union in those days was the closest thing you could get to a quick, electronic transfer of funds—but it wasn't all that quick.

I also called my friend Teena, who had comforted me a lot during the custody dispute. Her father had committed her mother to a mental institution—where she underwent shock therapy—for the seeming insanity of having an affair with another man. Teena was miserable living with her father, who wouldn't let her visit her mother. "She's not insane. He's just punishing her. I've got to get away from him," Teena said. "Why don't I go with you?"

Teena and I had been working together, cutting and pasting fine tissue paper to make multicolored lampshades that we intended to sell to craft shops. I suggested to Peter that we take Teena along. We could start a craft business in Arizona. We would achieve a balance of yin and yang at a charming country home in a beautiful green valley in Kingman. In our new life, we would be as free as peaceniks should be. We would avoid both the army and my family.

That evening while my parents were out playing bridge, Teena came by and we cabbed to LaGuardia Airport. I kept lookout through the car's back window. I was relieved to see nobody following us.

We had only twenty minutes before the flight's last call and rushed to buy tickets. When we alighted in Arizona, Ryan was waiting for us in the outdoor Arrivals area—there were no security gates back then. His eagle-beak nose shone reddish tan, and his blond hair had turned almost white. I thought he would be glad to see us, but stress wrinkled across his otherwise young face.

Della planted her feet on the ground, and I hugged Ryan. "You okay?" I asked.

"In a hurry," he said. "We've got to move out." He ushered the four of us through the terminal and into a beat-up Ford pickup truck. With Della on my lap, we squeezed into the cab. Warm air blew in through the windows. We passed clumps of cacti, stretches of brown and tan earth, and an occasional weathered shack. I looked for green grass and pretty streams, like the one in Ryan's picture. There were none.

"Everyone's at the house waiting for us, but we'll have to leave right away," Ryan said.

"Why?" Teena asked.

"Kingman doesn't like hippies."

"But I thought the house isn't in Kingman," I said.

"It is now."

Ryan explained that neighbors, unhappy that he and his friends lived communally, had come up with a strategy to get rid of them. The house butted the edge of town, so Kingman changed its boundaries. The commune was now within the dusty town. Ryan and his friends had to move out because the toilet was in an outhouse, and homes in Kingman were not allowed to have outhouses. Teena, Peter, Della, and I couldn't move in.

"They came yesterday and gave us twenty-four hours to get out," Ryan said.

"What happens if you don't leave?"

"They said they'd be happy to provide accommodations in jail."

I had been used to negative reactions to hippies in New York, but I had expected a more easygoing attitude out west. I was wrong. There was a stigma attached to being a hippie almost everywhere in America. Today the situation calls to mind the stigma attached to hepatitis C.

The car eventually stopped in front of a large, well-worn residence with gray-painted shingles. A Country Joe and the Fish concert poster, with text that drooped like an acid dream, was taped to the door. Ryan's four commune friends—three men and a woman—were piling possessions on the porch. It was obvious that we would need to find other lodgings. Few landlords, even in New York, would rent to a band of hippies, and the whole town of Kingman had turned against the commune. We needed to settle somewhere more agreeable. But we had only enough cash for groceries. Credit cards were rare at the time and probably not issued to hippies. Being homeless hadn't been part of the plan.

"What will we do?" I asked.

"We could go to Taos, New Mexico. There are some communes there," Teena said.

"We won't get far without money," Ryan said.

"I've got my pay coming," I said. "It should be at Western Union in a week. It should get us all to Taos."

"We'll camp for the week," Peter said.

Everyone perked up at the idea.

"Where's that stream you sent us the picture of? Can we camp there?" I asked Ryan.

"Sure, but I can't promise you the stream," he said, which was puzzling.

So the eight adults and a toddler piled into the Ford pickup, which belonged to Tommy, one of Ryan's friends. Della and I sat next to Tommy in the cab. He said he had grown up in Kingman. "My parents don't want me back home until I cut my hair," he said as the truck set off into the desert. "I won't do it."

I could understand why not. His shiny, sleek hair hung in a thick red ponytail past his shoulders.

The truck stopped at the bottom of a gravel road. We all got out and clambered down a short hill.

"This is the place," Ryan said, spreading his arms and twisting around to indicate an expanse of arid scenery.

The babbling stream surrounded by greenery and wildflowers he had captured in the photo was now a dry gully. There were no flowers. A few brown shrubs stood parched and nearly leafless. Cacti grew here and there with needlelike barbs sticking out. A lizard slithered past my foot. There were no flat areas. This wasn't a place to pitch a tent.

"Where do we camp?" asked Raccoon, whose scrunched-in face looked like a raccoon's.

"Follow me," Ryan said. Together there were nine of us: five men, three women, and a child. Tommy and blond, chubby Alice carried guitars. Greg, with the curly beard, carried bongos. As we walked, we sang songs, and the two groups got to know each other. We stopped for a water break and chatted about what we'd do in Taos. One of the communes Teena had heard of raised chickens and made crafts. Peter, Teena, and I were craftspeople, so that suited us well. Ryan and Raccoon could help with the chickens. Greg, Tommy, and Alice would build chicken coops.

We hiked about half a mile along a dusty trail onto a plateau above a dry but majestic canyon. On one side a craggy granite wall climbed straight up, about twice our height. Then it sloped more gently toward distant mountains. Below the plateau a shallow canyon snaked away from us.

We set up tents that the three Kingman hippies had brought from their homes. Peter, Tommy, and Greg hiked back to the truck and drove to the nearest store for supplies. They returned with two coolers of ice, several gallons of water, and bags of groceries. Tommy with his streaming red hair and Alice with her streaming blond hair tuned up their guitars, bongos appeared, and music erupted in the desert. The guitar players sang Beatles', Rolling Stones', Mamas and Papas', and Bee Gees' songs. Soon everyone in the group had learned all the lyrics to the songs, and everyone sang along. The bongos moved from person to person and the drumming style changed accordingly. We spent the next three days listening to music, singing, and eating huge meals of eggs and tacos, hamburger meat and tacos, beans and tacos, and cheese and tacos. Occasionally we'd go for hikes, or one of the Kingman hippies would identify desert fauna for us. I learned you could slice into a watermelon cactus and squeeze out water. You'd have to be careful about the spines.

Della played with stacking toys and blocks I had brought. Mostly, though, she practiced talking. Except for "ma" and "hi," her talk was babble, but she was rapidly learning the sounds and nuances of English. Often she would dance around and holler "loco saloo, loco saloo." I couldn't figure out what those words meant and thought they were just her favorite speechlike sounds that really meant nothing.

In the late afternoon on the third day in the desert, everyone gathered around the fire. We roasted hot dogs and stirred a pot of beans to be eaten on tacos. Della danced around. Tommy and Alice played the Beatles' "Rocky Raccoon." They played and sang that a lot because Raccoon was in our group. The lyrics told about Rocky Raccoon visiting a local saloon. Della piped up with "loco saloo, loco saloo." We laughed, and then we sang "Puff the Magic Dragon" to her. As the sky dimmed and the sun sank low in a tableau of oranges and pink, Della's eyes began to close, and I took her to my tent, where she was asleep within seconds, cocooned in a thin baby sleeping bag. The 110-degree daytime heat had cooled to a pleasant 80. The music by the campfire became soulful. Tommy and Alice played the haunting "Michael

Row the Boat Ashore," which was first sung by slaves in the U.S. South, and we all joined in.

Then, from around the corner of the granite rock, came shuffling sounds. The singing and guitar plucking stopped. Beams of light shot across the desert floor. The lights hit our eyes. Rifles stuck out from behind the bend of the rock and pointed our way.

CHAPTER 8

# STOCK AND OTHER TICKERS

AFTER THAT FIRST visit with Maria in 2014, I slid into racing mode. I believe hep C had made me sluggish during the last two years of my infection, but I was determined to banish the demon. The race was on for money. I had to find the dollars to pay for the best of the drugs.

There was a chance my medical plan or my husband's would cover the gold-plated treatment, but it was slight. Maria had explained that few insurers would pay for the Sovaldi-Galexos drug combination. I was leaving my job. I had signed resignation papers. The courses I taught had been assigned to other instructors. My medical plan, even if it would pay for the drugs, could run out before I finished treatment.

My husband said I should opt for the non-interferon treatment no matter what, even if we had to pay full price. We could forgo many years of vacations, he said. We could manage on a much smaller budget, just to free me of the infection. I am the budget keeper in the family. I looked at our bank accounts and couldn't convince myself we could get through our retirement years if we were to pay for the top-rated treatment. The last thing I wanted was to mortgage the house.

Maria had given me the phone numbers of two patient support programs: the Momentum Patient Assistance Program (Support Path in the U.S.), sponsored by Gilead, the maker of Sovaldi; and the Galexos: BioAdvance Patient Support Program, sponsored by Janssen Pharmaceuticals, the maker of Galexos. Both might pay for all or part of a patient's drug costs, depending on the person's income, Maria said. The programs also helped patients get approval from their health plans for their drugs. Maria advised that when I talked with a Momentum rep, I should ask specifically if they could help. She suggested that accessing the Galexos program could be easier because Allison Waithe, the patient representative, was "really nice."

First I called Momentum, and its representative asked for proof of income. That worried me. During the last few years, I had worked as much as possible despite pain, flagging energies, and a muddled mind. My husband also worked at a college. Our family income looked good but was destined to dip severely soon. The rep said it would take a couple of days to determine where I stood in Momentum's subsidy scale. A couple of days felt like torture to my hep-frenzied mind, so I called Allison, the Galexos program rep. In the first of many phone calls with her, I learned she was as nice as Maria had said she was. A native of Trinidad, she responded to my questions with a mix of Canadian English and the reggae-song accent that's common in the Caribbean. She was always ready with a chuckle, and she had a knack of making me laugh even though I was worried about my health.

When I told her I had probably contracted hep C through a postpartum transfusion, she said, "My gosh, I didn't know you got it that way."

Allison's job included helping people through the maze of provincial drug plans and extended health insurance. Her job title was Reimbursement Specialist for the Galexos program (her company no longer holds that contract). The program provided subsidies for people who needed help with the cost of hepatitis C drugs.

I was relieved that it took less than a day for Allison to investigate the possible ways I could pay for my drugs. When I first talked with her, in July 2014, British Columbia's Fair PharmaCare Plan was yet to cover the direct-acting antivirals Dr. Ramji had prescribed. So Allison contacted my husband's medical plan, Manulife, and mine, Pacific Blue Cross. The next morning, she called back and said Al's plan wouldn't cover me, but my plan would. Most extended medical plans at the time paid only for drugs approved under PharmaCare, but Blue Cross's policy with my employer paid for all prescription drugs.

During the six days between my visit with Dr. Ramji and the beginning of treatment, I spent at least twenty-five hours talking on the phone, emailing, filling out forms, and, twice, taking a ferry to visit my insurance company, all in a frantic effort to make sure my drugs would be paid for. Otherwise, they might not arrive. The pharmacy would deliver them directly to my home but required payment before they were shipped. My extended medical plan had agreed to fund the drugs, but the insurance company wanted me to pay first and they would reimburse me later. I could pay only by credit card but was worried I'd get stuck with hefty interest charges. I was told I could send the insurer an assignment of payment form so that they could pay the pharmacy directly. There were complications and delays with that, so I tried to pay on credit.

For the first shipment, I would get a one-month supply of Galexos and Sovaldi, which cost approximately $38,000. I had three credit cards. I could max them out to come up with the cash, but each had a different maximum. There's the adage that when something can go wrong, it usually does. And it did. One party even got my name wrong, so a new form had to be filled out in all of its check-box and please-print intricacy. Forms had to be faxed, not emailed, when few people still owned fax machines. The wrong amounts were charged to the credit cards, and my cards went over their limit. I had to get refunds and start from square one with the credit charges. The problems were all human errors; I was told someone new had been working in billing. The pharmacy was very nice and forthcoming, the insurance company was very nice and forthcoming, and I was stressed out.

Hepatitis C has always been expensive to cure or even to try to cure, but the notion of "expensive" is subjective. In the year 2000 in the United States, the average cost of treatment with interferon plus ribavirin, laboratory testing, and visits to the doctor gobbled up $10,000 to $12,000. Dozens of medical researchers debated the cost effectiveness of the drugs. Since then the price of a cure for hepatitis C has climbed so high that $10,000 seems like turkey feed.

Alpha interferon was approved for use against hep C in 1991, just as doctors had begun to recognize hep C as a distinct virus and not just a "non-A, non-B" liver infection. Back then, alpha interferon had to be injected three times a week.

It took eight years before the antiviral ribavirin was added. In 2001 the pegylated variety of interferon came on the market and reduced the weekly injections to one. The cure rate of 44 percent with interferon alone increased to about 60 percent when ribavirin and pegylated interferon were combined. (Some studies cite the cure rate as up to 80 percent, depending on genotype.) The $10,000 treatment with awful side effects remained the standard for another decade. Some people with hep C who couldn't afford or were afraid of the treatment turned to healthy foods and naturopathy to ward off their disease. Although the natural route was generally cheaper and much easier on the body than interferon, there was no significant evidence that it provided a cure. Doctors continued to prescribe interferon.

On Monday, July 7, 2014, Health Canada released a decision allowing the use of the first non-interferon, non-ribavirin treatment for hepatitis C. I met with Dr. Ramji three days later, and he prescribed the combo for me. When I heard about the cost—and learned that if I couldn't pay it, I would probably have to take interferon and get horrendously sick—money issues jumped ahead of the disease on my worry list. But I was lucky I lived in Canada. South of the border, the total cost of the two drugs would be near $150,000 in U.S. dollars. That was about $30,000 U.S. more than the Canadian price during a month when the Canadian dollar traded at about 93 cents U.S. Using a historical currency converter I found on the web, I calculated an actual $47,390 Cdn. difference between the prices.

One of the reasons for the lower price in Canada is that drug prices there go through the Patented Medicine Prices Review Board (PMPRB). Canada changed its Patent Act in 1987 to allow pharmaceutical companies exclusive rights to their medicines for twenty years, up from seventeen. The

Progressive Conservative government said the change would encourage drug companies to invest in new drug research in Canada. To rein in drug manufacturers that might charge exorbitant prices during the longer patenting period, the government set up the review board. The PMPRB states on its website that it ensures "that the prices of patented medicines sold in Canada are not excessive." The board determines excessiveness by comparing Canadian drug prices with the cost of drugs in Germany, France, Italy, Sweden, Switzerland, the UK, and, oddly, the number one country for astronomical drug costs, the United States. It then uses a formula to ensure that Canadians pay no more than the median price. It may issue orders to drug companies to lower their prices. Nonetheless, a median price among excessive prices is still excessive.

Odder still is that the cost of the new hep C drugs varies wildly from country to country and from patient to patient, which makes it difficult to nail down prices. Gilead Sciences seems to price Sovaldi at whatever the market will bear. That varies a lot according to market segment. In Egypt and Brazil at the time of my treatment, patients paid just $840 U.S. for three months of the drug. Kenyans and Iranians paid only $900. In the U.S. the cost was a hundred times higher: $94,000. In a capitalist economy, this kind of pricing makes sense to shareholders when there are no competitors for a product. That's good and fine when a teen is desperate for an iPhone. However, the median wealth in the United States was less than half of the cost of Sovaldi ($44,900 in August 2014), and the median household income just $53,046, according to the 2013 census. This made a lot of patients nervous about the cost of the treatment they desperately needed. Some people in the U.S. were wealthy or lucky enough to have a gold-plated insurance plan, or they were poor and sick enough to have the state pay the bill. For everyone else, the miracle cure was unaffordable.

Gilead's strategy included heavy discounts for countries that insisted on heavy discounts, discounts for government departments that insisted on discounts, discounts for medical plans and HMOs, and a support program that would subsidize people who couldn't afford their insurance deductible. In 2016, insurance companies in the U.S. were getting about a 45 percent discount off the cost of Sovaldi,[1] which helped increase purchases of the drug—for some insured people. GILD shares on the NASDAQ exchange doubled in price between the year before and the year after my treatment. By February 2015, sales of Sovaldi and of Gilead's newer hepatitis C drug, Harvoni, totaled $12.4 billion.

Gilead took a lot of flak from the media about the price of Sovaldi. Around the time I began my treatment, the U.S. Senate began an investigation into the $1,000-per-pill drug. Not only was the medication expensive for patients, but it also had the potential to hammer the government's health care programs. The Veterans Health Administration was concerned. State Medicaid programs were alarmed. On April 8, 2015, the *Wall Street Journal* reported that the previous year, Medicaid programs had spent $1.33 billion on hepatitis drugs. Most of that was for Sovaldi, which was the highest-priced treatment in 2014. The next year Harvoni, which combined Sovaldi with another Gilead-developed direct-acting antiviral, jumped to the top in sales.

Medicaid, run individually by each U.S. state, subsidizes health care costs for the poor. The Patient Protection and Affordable Care Act, passed under President Barack Obama, stated that anyone whose income falls below 133 percent of the poverty line could receive Medicaid, but after the bill's passage, the Supreme Court ruled that states needn't agree to this income line. Hard-pressed public health care providers couldn't afford to pay for treatment for everyone with HCV. In just nine months in 2014, states forked over more than $1.08 billion for Sovaldi (sofosbuvir), one of the two drugs I used. They paid $136.3 million for the other part of my two-pill treatment. States receive at least a 23.1 percent rebate of the drug cost under law, so some of the money may have gone back into the system.

Nonetheless, the price remained too high, so states developed rationing plans for direct-acting antivirals. The line was most often drawn at stage 3 liver damage, with almost everyone below that level receiving no treatment. In one state—Texas—no patient received state-paid treatment. It was just too expensive for the legislature's liking. In April 2015, the state relented somewhat and began paying for AbbVie's Viekira Pak, a multi-pill regimen that was less expensive than the Gilead drugs, for patients with advanced liver disease.

Another cost-reduction tactic was to threaten or take legal action. In early 2016, Massachusetts's attorney general sent a letter to Gilead asking that its hep C drug prices be lowered. China got into the fray by refusing Gilead a patent on Sovaldi. That would allow China to manufacture its own sofosbuvir, which would be a substantial bargain. A study of mass manufacturing costs estimated that the drug could be produced for less than $2 a pill.[2] But pricing for patients in developed countries continued at hundreds of times more than that.

In early 2016, Gilead was charging $94,500 U.S. for a twelve-week course of its one-pill hep C miracle cure, Harvoni. On January 28, 2016, the U.S. Food and Drug Administration (FDA) approved the Merck drug Zepatier for genotypes 1 and 4. Canadian approval came the next month for genotypes 1, 3, and 4. The treatment was listed at $54,600 in the U.S., giving Gilead big competition for a once-a-day, one-pill, twelve-week miracle cure. Gilead came back with another one-pill-a-day miracle cure, Epclusa, which the FDA approved in the summer of 2016. At around $75,000 for a twelve-week treatment, Epclusa cures all major genotypes, 1 to 6. Patients today have a choice of several hep C drugs. Here's where the prices stood in spring through summer of 2016:

- Viekira Pak (Holkira Pak in Canada) from AbbVie Inc., at $83,000 U.S. for three tablets a day for twelve weeks.
- Harvoni from Gilead, which supplanted Gilead's own drug Sovaldi, as well as Janssen's Galexos, with a one-pill treatment at $94,500 for twelve weeks.
- Daklinza, used to treat genotype 3, a drug-resistant strain of hepatitis C that harms the liver faster than the other genotypes. Bristol-Myers Squibb received FDA approval for the drug in July 2015 and priced it at $63,000 for a twelve-week treatment. It's combined with $84,000 worth of Sovaldi for a total cost of $147,000 in the United States. That soon became way too expensive to be competitive. In August 2016 I found coupons on the Web for Daklinza from U.S. pharmacies, including Walgreens, CVS, Walmart, and Target. All offered at least a 33 percent discount. The best discount coupon was for Kmart, which offered $22,319.20 off the price of the drug.
- Technivie, from the pharmaceutical company AbbVie, approved for genotype 4 around the same time as Daklinza. The drug is used for twelve weeks with ribavirin. The initial cost was $76,653 for twelve weeks.
- Zepatier, a combination of grazoprevir and elbasvir, for

which Merck received FDA approval in January 2016. The once-daily pill treats genotypes 1 and 4 without ribavirin. The list price was $54,600 U.S. for a twelve-week treatment, making it at the time the least costly of the non-interferon direct-acting antivirals for hepatitis C. That was good for patients' budgets, at least for those with the requisite genotypes whose dollars could stretch that far.

Then came Epclusa. It was approved by the FDA in June 2016, and by the UK and Canada the next month. The $74,760 treatment combines Sovaldi and the NS5A inhibitor velpatasvir. It showed a 98 percent cure rate and could eliminate the need for genotype testing, and it would help people who suffered from the least curable types of hep. Millions of people would want the new cure. That would assure increasing dividends for Gilead, I reasoned as I considered buying GILD shares. I opened an Internet stock ticker and noted the pronounced hump in Gilead's graph. Yet I felt uneasy about investing. Hep C drugs were being rationed because of their costs, and the costs were preposterous because shareholders clamored for profits. My hippie distaste for uncontrolled capitalism rushed back to me. My finger was poised to press the "buy" button, but I pulled away.

BETWEEN MY FIRST visit with Dr. Ramji and the day I was slated to receive my drugs, I needed two more blood tests. One was a baseline PCR test, which would show my viral load at the start of treatment. The other was a blood panel that would help determine the state of my liver. These blood panel indicators, among more than two dozen that were tested, are commonly looked at in relation to hepatitis C:

- AST (aspartate aminotransferase) is an enzyme that is released into the bloodstream when internal body tissues are damaged. AST can build up in organs such as the heart, the brain, and the liver. A higher than normal AST level might indicate hepatitis, but it could also rise when someone is having a heart attack or muscle injury.
- ALT (alanine aminotransferase) is concentrated in the liver, works in the liver, and normally stays in the liver. When the liver is scarred, ALT may leak into the bloodstream and create elevated levels there.
- Bilirubin is the yellow substance that causes jaundice. It comes from the breakdown of hemoglobin, the iron-containing protein in red blood cells. From the liver, bilirubin moves into the colon and out of the body. If the bile ducts are blocked because of hepatitis, bilirubin levels may rise.

A few days later I looked at my test results online. I was happy to see close to normal enzyme levels. I would have to get blood taken once a week during my treatment, but that was okay. I had gotten used to being a pincushion.

My main concern was whether my drugs were on their way. Until the day—or actually the minute—my drugs arrived, I wasn't totally convinced they were coming. In the few days since Dr. Ramji had prescribed the treatment, there had been mixed messages and screw-ups about payment for the first month's supply. The combination of Sovaldi and Galexos would cost $38,000 for just the first four weeks out of twelve. In paying for that first month, I stretched my cards to, and accidentally over, the limit. I would be reimbursed later by my extended health plan, but not without stress about the whopping interest the cards charged for lateness.

Around this time Adam Bailey was also worried about paying for direct-acting antivirals. Adam was a friend of a good friend of mine, and like me he had recently learned he was infected with hepatitis C.

When Adam was in his twenties, he played guitar in a rock band. On evenings when he didn't have a gig, he'd get together with his buddies at someone's home. They'd have a few beers, listen to music, and talk. One time he and his friends watched in amazement as a group of people injected themselves with cocaine. "It looked like they were having fun," Adam said. Another evening, as someone dissolved white powder in water on a spoon, Adam held out his arm. Over the next couple of weeks he may have pierced his arm a few more times, but he's not sure. He snorted a lot of coke back then, and his memories of the time are fuzzy.

About a month after his first experiment with injected cocaine, Adam found a girlfriend. She became and still is his wife. "She was not into that sort of thing [cocaine]," he said. Adam began to think about a future including kids. He ended his coke days then and there. More than three decades later, he learned he was infected with hepatitis C.

I visited Adam at his home on a hillside near Squamish, British Columbia. He and his wife had just celebrated their thirtieth anniversary. They have two kids, a boy and a girl, and the boy has two kids, a boy and a girl. I parked near the driveway of Adam's freshly mowed quarter-acre property and marveled at the serenity of the neighborhood. As I knocked on the door Adam hollered, "Just a minute. Just a minute. The door's open. Come in." I entered the tidy, high-ceilinged, open-plan home and found him scrubbing at tiles along the kitchen counter. He pointed toward the gray-smudged ceiling. "I just walked out of the room and didn't notice something burning on the stove," he said as he scoured the smoky residue.

In a black T-shirt, slim black pants, and black boots, Adam still looked like a rocker. He exudes a Steven Tyler–like persona and is wiry like the Aerosmith singer too. His spiky gray hair and the deep creases from his mouth to his cheekbones were the only signs he had reached age fifty-seven. Otherwise, he appeared at least fifteen years younger.

Adam learned he had antibodies to the hep C virus in 2013. His next test revealed that the disease was chronic. "It was a shock for me. I run and I work out, and I eat well," he said. "I was surprised to hear that number one, I had been exposed, and number two, that I had active hepatitis."

Adam is among the majority of hep C patients in Canada and the United States whose infection may have begun while injecting intravenous drugs (cited at 61 percent of hep C patients in 2010). When he experimented with cocaine, he felt he was being adventurous. Adam's infection, like my hepatitis C infection, like everyone's hepatitis C infection, was an accident.

Despite the enormous changes in his life, Adam was coming to grips with the results of his rock 'n' roll youth. His doctor had given him a choice, much like the one I had faced. He could be treated with easy direct-acting antivirals or endure the old standard, interferon.

"I really don't want to take this interferon," he told me.

At that time all but one genotype had to be treated with at least some of the older drug in combination with the new antivirals. (My genotype—the somewhat rare 1b—had just become the exception.) Adam's doctor had suggested sofosbuvir (Sovaldi) plus interferon, which would cut his treatment from forty-eight weeks down to twelve. But first, the doctor said, Adam needed a liver biopsy. Adam didn't like the idea of somebody stabbing him in the gut.

I explained how a FibroScan works. I suggested he ask his doctor if he could have one instead of a biopsy. "But don't worry," I said, adding that another friend with hep C, Ben Handley, had gone through a liver biopsy. "They do put a needle in," I said. "Apparently it's pretty small and they use a local anesthetic. My friend said it wasn't a big deal."

Adam said he would probably get the biopsy. Even if it hurt, it was a necessary step before treatment, according to his doctor, and Adam wanted desperately to be treated. It had been over a year since he was diagnosed, and the demon was swimming through his body and his consciousness.

"The worst part of this whole thing is that it's always, always on, every waking minute in my mind," he said. "Every time you feel a headache or any kind of ailment at all, your mind says, is this it?"

I still felt that way, too—up until and beyond the day I started treatment. It was as if someone were holding a gun to my head. For all I knew, it would go off. It was like that day in the desert when the posse came.

## July 1969, Night

# POSSE

SEVEN MEN EMERGED from behind the massive rock that formed the backdrop of our campsite. Cowboy boots tromped over dusty ground, kicking at saltbush and purple-flowered sage. Each of the men held a gun. Most carried rifles, but a couple of them gripped pistols. We backed away, raising our hands. The men motioned for us to form a line in front of them.

The sheriff, wearing a star-shaped badge, shuffled to the front. He said we had to leave the desert and leave Kingman. "You're breaking the law, and we're here to enforce it," he said.

"What law?" Ryan asked.

"You're trespassing."

"On the desert?"

"On the desert! This is not your property! Get moving. You have three minutes to pack up and get moving," the sheriff said, motioning with his rifle toward the far side of the rock.

I sprinted to my tent and scooped up Della. A few of the men, probably not expecting a child to be present, gaped at me. We frantically pulled down tents and stuffed everything we could as quickly as possible in bags and coolers. The posse signaled us to follow them. They all had flashlights, but we had found only a few in the jumble of our belongings before we were told to march into the growing darkness.

The Mohave spreads through the driest region of California, Nevada, Utah, and Arizona and supports thousands of plant species. As we set off on a long, forced trek while night settled in, it seemed like all of them were cacti. They blended into the gray nighttime sand and stabbed me as I passed— I had foolishly worn shorts. Barrel cacti that brightened the desert with orange, cuplike flowers during the day lost many spines to my legs that night. Spanish dagger plants sliced my shins. I held Della closely, alert for prickly things in the night.

We plodded through the desert, at first two by two and then single file as we entered a narrow path along the gulch where Ryan's pretty stream had once flowed. The sky was turning black with a sprinkle of stars. The posse men gabbed with each other about hunting, politics in the town, and how longhairs were destroying society. My friends and I said nothing. All I could think of was that the men who were herding us carried guns. Three were at the front of the line, and the other four brought up the rear.

I hugged Della close most of the way, but occasionally I would stumble over a rock or wince from a cactus stab. Teena, behind me, would take my daughter for a minute or two while I regained equilibrium. Della was quiet through it all, fluttering her eyes now and then. The desert air had chilled. My legs were getting cold and more and more scratched from the cacti.

Eventually the men in front shone their flashlights onto a paved road in front of us. A car and a pickup truck stood in the dirt.

"Who's from around here?" the sheriff asked.

Tommy, Greg, and Alice stepped forward. The sheriff directed them with his rifle into the back of the car. Three of the posse men got into the front.

"The rest of you, in there," he said, pointing to the back of the pickup. Peter, Ryan, Teena, Raccoon, and I shoved the few possessions we had been able to rescue into the box and climbed in. One of the posse men clambered in with us. He held his gun on his lap, which kept us quiet as the truck started up and moved onto the highway. The car with our Kingman friends followed for a while but soon turned onto a dark minor road. That was the last I saw of those gentle desert hippies. Soon the truck stopped alongside a sidewalk in town. Peter, Ryan, Teena, Raccoon, and I, with Della in my arms, filed into the police station.

I had visions of being thrown into jail or standing in front of a judge or both. The sheriff told my New York contingent and Raccoon, who was from Chicago, to wait on a bench in the hallway. We waited. I watched the slim red second hand of a big wall clock sweep around thick gray numbers. After six hours, it was 5 a.m.

I craved sleep. My head sank onto my chest. A voice hollered, "Up! Stand up!"

Two deputies led us outside and prodded us toward the back of a pickup truck (it seemed like almost everyone in Arizona drove a pickup). "We want you out of this town," one of the deputies said. We climbed into the truck bed. The engine groaned. We were heading out of Kingman and into the desert. The sun broke through wispy clouds. The truck stopped on Route I-40 in the middle of nowhere.

"Get out!" the driver said. We climbed out of the back of the pickup with our paltry belongings. Everything we owned except a half-filled duffel bag and my bag of baby things had been left at our campsite or thrown into the trunk of the car that took our Kingman friends.

"Where should we go?" Teena asked.

"Just go! Don't come back!" He slammed his door shut and drove off.

Our little group sat together by the side of the road on desert dust and stones. Della woke and seemed happy with our location. The rest of us weren't.

WE DEBATED HANGING around for a few more days and sneaking into town to collect my paycheck. We counted the few dollars we were carrying. There was barely enough for one night at a motel for all of us. And there would be nowhere we could stay near the town without attracting the attention of the posse.

"Well, due east is Santa Fe," Raccoon said, scrunching his mouth the way he often did. "We could hitchhike there."

We all agreed to hitch to New Mexico. We decided to split into two groups so it would be easier to get a ride. We would meet in the Santa Fe bus station and take the bus from there to Taos, where people like us who accepted people like us would welcome us. There were six of us, including my daughter. I said my group should have an extra adult to make sure she was okay. Peter, Ryan, and I, holding Della, stayed put and stuck out our thumbs. Teena and Raccoon marched down the hill behind us waving and singing.

After a while a car passed us by.

A car passed us by.

A car passed us by.

A camper was passing us. Teena and Raccoon hung out its back window, grinned at us, and waved. We waved back. The camper passed us by.

A car passed us by.

A truck passed us by.

A car passed us by.

It was July in the desert. The wispy clouds dissipated. The temperature climbed. I pulled out a water bottle from the baby bag and passed it around. The sun above looked ominous. Nobody had a watch, but time ticked away.

# PART III

*BANISHMENT*

## CHAPTER 9

# A LETTER

T IME TICKED AND ticked into my hepatitis summer, but I didn't feel much closer to getting treatment. On Saturday, the day after my blood tests, two days after I had met with Dr. Ramji, and four days before the two components of my miracle cure were set to arrive—if, and only if, I could pay for them—each second seemed like an eternity. I woke early and stumbled toward the kitchen. My eyes were red and itchy. I had hardly slept, and my nerves jangled more than usual because of the financial wrangling I'd been doing to pay for the drugs. Zeena's chocolate eyes stared at me wistfully, pleading for breakfast. I fed her, and then it was time for a walk.

With Zeena off leash and following me, I hiked up the steep, shady driveway. Brush, tangles of blackberry vines, and overhanging tree boughs ended at the top of the slope. From there to the community mailbox, the road lay flat and bathed in sun. My funky mood was clearing. I was beginning to feel confident that I would get the drugs I needed.

And they'd cure me, I was nearly sure. I opened my cubby in the mailbox and pulled out a letter. It was from the office of Dr. Louise Halliman.

She must have received notice of my HCV infection, I thought. This is probably a letter of sympathy and an apology for not detecting it. The letter had come just when I was most worried, and it would certainly cheer me up. I decided that the next time I was in Vancouver I would stop by her office and invite her for coffee.

When I got back home I opened the envelope. There wasn't much to read:

Service for chart summary and transfer of medical records: $25.00

Two days later, the pharmacy confirmed it would be delivering the drugs directly to my home. The payment method for that first shipment remained uncertain, but I could forgo my next new car if need be. Two days after that, the day before my clinic appointment, I waited for the drugs to arrive.

My daughter Della waited with me. So did my friend Jen, one of the few people I had so far told about my illness. We lounged in the sun on my patio, drinking lots of tea. My companions asked about my illness and from time to time changed the subject to something less stressful, and then I'd say something about my illness and we'd start talking about it again. It felt wonderful having my wonderful daughter stay with me during this vigil. Having a wonderful friend there as well was a bonus. They calmed me as much as I *could* be calmed.

Periodically I'd excuse myself and trot up the driveway to see if the delivery truck was on its way. I would be traveling to the GI clinic in Vancouver the next day, and Maria had asked that I bring the pills to her office. I absolutely needed those pills. But a lot had gone wrong so far. I waited and waited, growing more nervous by the hour. In the late afternoon Della had to catch the ferry to be with my grandkids. I saw her off, returned to the deck, and waited with Jen.

It was the end of the business day. I feared the truck may have already come and gone from the neighborhood without delivering my shipment. It was hard to find my driveway amid the vines, maples, and cedar trees that cloaked it. My house was hidden too. Many delivery trucks in the past had given up hunting for my address. To help the drug truck find it, I had posted signs with bold black arrows on yellow paper onto a tree and a shed. But those could be missed as well.

When Jen was leaving, I took another jaunt up the driveway to the road. At the top a truck was making a U-ey. "Wait! Wait!" I hollered, and I scrambled to the driver's door. He stopped and handed me a white box and a clipboard with a document to sign.

I carried the box into the house as if it were made of the thinnest filigreed glass. It was the size of a hatbox with two-inch walls of dense Styrofoam. I pulled up the lid. Two plastic prescription bottles rested among chilled gel packs; the pills needed to stay at 59–86 degrees F, and I was worried about them losing their strength. It was the hottest day of summer so far, with the thermometer climbing above 90. I had to keep the treasure cool.

THAT SAME DAY, my niece Sandy was trying to get treatment for hepatitis C. Sandy was on Medicaid in Florida, which had denied her treatment with the new drugs. My sister Mary, Sandy's mother, called me and asked about clinical trials that provide drugs free to patients. I said I'd browse for one on the Internet. I couldn't find a trial anywhere in Florida that would take Sandy. At the time, my genotype, 1b, was the only one being treated without interferon. Sandy had genotype 1a, so the best she could hope for was Sovaldi plus interferon for twelve weeks. Her doctor refused to prescribe interferon because it tends to depress people, and Sandy had endured episodes of depression.

Sandy, who's about ten years younger than I am, has reason to be depressed at times. Besides the hep, she is prone to severe acid reflux, which has sent her to the hospital twice. Her teeth have rotted from poor nutrition. A tumor has grown on her pituitary gland, causing Cushing's syndrome, which raises cortisol levels in the blood, which leads to weight gain. Over nine months, Sandy's weight rocketed from 138 pounds to 215. She suffers from foot pain and at times can hardly walk. Yet I think she would gladly keep any of these problems, including the hep, if she could get rid of her most troubling affliction, schizophrenia. I speculated that the makers of the new antivirals had little interest in targeting people like Sandy, who were unlikely to have incomes that could pay the price of the drugs.

Later that year, I visited my sister Mary and we drove to Sandy's home, a plain but pleasant-looking rancher on a winding lane amid a palm-spotted tract of similar ranchers in Ocala, Florida. To my surprise, Sandy recognized me. I hadn't seen her for more than twenty-five years. We all decided to go out for lunch. As we were getting into Mary's car, Sandy handed her mother a bag of Hershey's bars and another of Reese's Peanut Butter Cups. "These are for you. I love you, Mom," she said.

Sandy is sturdily built and looks healthy, with glowing cheeks and glossy black hair as thick as a Samoyed's, which she had set back from her face with bobby pins. I remarked that the style was lovely, and Sandy smiled. She is a gentle, gracious woman when she's on her meds. But occasionally she goes off of them. If she forgets them once, she's less likely to take the next dose, Mary explained. Then everything goes awry.

That doesn't happen these days because Sandy lives with a certified nursing assistant. Barbara truly cares for Sandy and hangs out with her when my sister can't be there. Previously, Barbara worked in a group home, looking after Sandy and several other psychotic adults. All except Sandy were unruly. Even when they stuck to their meds they were hard to control. Mary recalled a time she volunteered to take the group to a park in central Florida for a hike. "They'd all go 'I don't want to hike there,' or 'I don't like it here,'" Mary said. Sandy was the only one who agreed to the proposed plans. Between her caregiver and her mother, Sandy's support system is solid.

Sandy pored over a colorful plastic-covered menu at the Steak 'n Shake restaurant in Ocala. "Could I please have a Coke, a Diet Coke?" she asked in her low-volume, deep-toned voice.

Mary responded, "Yes you may, Sweetie."

Mary and I placed our orders, and I noticed Sandy averting her eyes and muttering to herself. "She's talking to God," Mary said.

Sandy contracted hep C in the 1980s in California. She was beset with hallucinations and living in homeless squalor. Sometime back then she acquired a tattoo, a peacock that spreads across her back just under her shoulder. Mary believes it was the source of the hep. Transmission of the hepatitis C virus through tattoos is rare in clean tattoo parlors. When friends or prisoners use unsterilized tattooing equipment, however, the risk rises to 2.0 to 3.6 percent, according to researchers from the Centers for Disease Control and Prevention in Atlanta.

Sandy returned to her family in Florida in 2001, sporting the tattoo and raving about nonsense. Mary took her to a psychiatrist, who treated Sandy for schizophrenia. Today "Sandy is a sweet, gentle girl when she's on her meds," said Mary. "Sandy's a different person when she's off her meds. She's belligerent. She's a paranoid schizophrenic. She thinks everybody's trying to kill her."

No one was taking away those meds, but there were other meds she needed. She had a biopsy that showed stage 2 fibrosis.

The specialist refused to treat Sandy because interferon might conflict with her antipsychotics and lead to depression. Mary next visited another doctor, who said he would treat the hep with permission from Sandy's psychiatrist. The psychiatrist wouldn't agree. Then the new antivirals came along. By the summer of 2015 Sandy's doctor had approved Harvoni for her. Sandy's problem shifted from getting a doctor's consent to getting money to pay for the drugs. In 2016 she was still waiting.

So I was amazingly lucky compared with Sandy. It took merely two months from the day I was diagnosed to the day I received my miracle drugs. The two little opaque white containers had been delivered, boxed and cushioned among gel packs. Inside one of the containers were twenty-eight white capsules of Galexos (simeprevir). Inside the other were twenty-eight tan, football-shaped tablets of Sovaldi (sofosbuvir). Maria had asked me to bring the entire one-month pill supply to her office.

I drove onto the ferry at six in the morning with close to $40,000 worth of prescription drugs in my purse, which I placed carefully on the passenger seat. I stayed in my red Toyota Echo during the sailing, fearing that the precious prescription would get lost, be stolen, or accidentally drop over the rail into the ocean if I ventured onto the upper deck. Or I might fling them over the rail myself—not because I didn't desperately want to start treatment, but because I was so nervous, my brain seemed to be shaking loose.

With the purse strap secured around my shoulder and the purse held tightly to my chest, I entered the office tower that housed the GI Research Institute. During the brief ride up on the elevator I watched two women and a man. The women spoke with each other and the man glanced my way. Maybe he suffered from hep, couldn't afford the pills, and knew what I was carrying. Even a non-thief, when desperate, might be tempted to grab the precious pills. I told myself that was silly, but I was still on edge from the demon. Finally I made it through the clinic's door, down the narrow hallway, and into the treatment lounge.

I pulled the little bottles from my purse and gave them to Maria. She passed me a container of yogurt, saying I might need something in my stomach before I downed the pills.

We talked as I ate. I asked questions about the future of my treatment, and the topic of my baseline PCR test came up.

"What was the count?" I asked, expecting the viral load to be about the same as last time, twenty thousand.

"One hundred and seventy-six thousand."

"What?" I must have turned white.

Maria said not to worry. "Sometimes it happens. It can go up and down."

Andrew Loog Oldham, the former manager of the Rolling Stones, learned in the late 1990s, soon after being diagnosed with hepatitis C, that he had a viral load of 4 million. He had freed himself of drug dependency by exercising and eating healthy food. About fifteen years later his count was down to 1.3 million. My viral load just after diagnosis had been a mere 20,000. I too ate healthy food and exercised. But two months later the count had jumped almost ninefold to 176,000 hepatitis C RNA particles in every milliliter of my blood. I did the math: The human body contains about 5 liters of blood, which equals 5,000 milliliters. I'm a small person, so my body would hold less. A 176,000 count for 3.5-liter me meant I had more than 600 million bits of the demon surging through my body.

At the institute that day my peace of mind, already in pieces over my disease, was shattered into 176,000 bits. It seemed like my hep was exploding. I wondered if the cutting-edge cure I was to be starting that day could possibly work while the virus writhed through my system in a reproductive orgy.

"It's still very low," Maria said.

Viral load has little to do with how quickly you develop symptoms of hepatitis C or liver scarring. Rather, the numbers relate to the prognosis for treatment. The higher your load of HCV particles, the longer it usually takes to be cured. (Although today, with direct-acting antivirals, cures are quick for almost anyone.) Conversely, the lower the load, the greater the chance you will achieve sustained virologic response quickly. Viral loads can go as high as the tens of millions. Researchers have pegged a low viral count as 800,000 or less. Nonetheless, on that first day of treatment I wondered what I might have done, or what the demon had done, to ramp up my infection. Maybe my age was catching up with my hep. But I was lucky it caught up when it did, rather than earlier. In fact, in a way I was lucky my infection with hepatitis C hadn't been detected earlier. Even a week or two sooner might have propelled me into interferon treatment.

I passed the empty yogurt container and spoon to Maria, and she passed me a can of passion-fruit juice. She opened the Sovaldi bottle and shook out one of the pills. As she placed it in my palm, she said, "Better not drop it. That's a thousand bucks."

The tension broke. I laughed, downed the Sovaldi with some juice and then the Galexos.

I went home to the Sunshine Coast. The next day was the second day of treatment and my first day of downing the pills without support. That may sound strange. What able-throated person needs support in swallowing pills? But I needed psychological support. I could feel those demons, which had turned into mechanical roly-poly bugs in my mind. I had seen a lot of drawings of the symmetrical virus. I now imagined HCV as nano-balls of spiky metal, scratching and screeching through my liver.

My husband had left for work at six in the morning, and I was alone in the living room watching the sunrise cast orangy pink ripples onto the ocean. Almost nothing could be more beautiful, but few days could find me more anxious. The two tablets I was to take each day for twelve weeks had to be swallowed at the same time every day. I would be getting a total of $115,000 worth of medication. I worried about the 15 percent chance of failure (as stated by Dr. Ramji; the drug companies' test results were much better). I figured some of the failures occurred because patients ignored the directions for optimum efficacy of the drugs. In other words, some people may have forgotten to swallow their pills on time. I decided my ideal time each day would be 7:30 a.m., when I was always awake and had the fewest distractions. I would make sure to take the pills then, no matter what.

I designed an Excel chart, which I printed and hung on my refrigerator. It had check boxes for the 7:30 a.m. daily pill-taking and also boxes to check off my weekly viral load tests, my hematology panels every two weeks, calls I needed to make to Allison or Maria, and my doctor's appointments. I rummaged through the "everything" drawer in the kitchen. I grabbed black and red indelible markers and a ruler, and I drew a pill-taking chart on the lid of the Styrofoam box the pills had come in. I placed the two bottles of pills on top of the lid. I also taped a mercury weather thermometer on top of it. I'd check the reading a few times in the warm part of the day to make sure the pills stayed in the recommended temperature range. The box lid and paraphernalia sat in the center of my kitchen island for the whole three months of my treatment. I would take my medicine at the correct time each day. I would tick off the boxes on the chart. I would follow the doctor's directions to the letter no matter what.

It was 7:30 a.m.; I swallowed the second set of pills. Then I composed a letter to Dr. Halliman, telling her I had been diagnosed with hepatitis C. I wrote that I believed she knew about it because her name was on the requisition for my hep C liver ultrasound. I typed and typed, projecting my indignation at the computer screen, making hard clacks on the keyboard. I told the doctor I had intended to invite her to lunch so we could talk as friends, but I was too disappointed to do so now. Next I wrote:

"Here's the check for $25."

The letter meandered into a rant about the money issue. I couldn't stop worrying that my fight with the virus might drain my retirement fund. It was only the second day of treatment, and side effects could occur. With interferon they often appeared weeks into the drug-taking. If that were to happen with my drug combo, would the possibility of a cure be worth the woe?

During the next few days the only physical side effect I felt from the two pills I took each morning was a minor stomach upset. I would nibble a handful of Goldfish crackers, and the heaviness in my gut would dissipate in twenty minutes. The upset stomach after pill-taking was much milder than I had experienced with antibiotics or Tylenol, and nerves rather than meds may have caused it. In less than a week after the first day of treatment, the discomfort vanished. After that, there were no physical side effects. That surprised me, especially since simeprevir, half of my regimen, could irritate the eyes or cause photosensitivity to the point of blistering after a short time in the sun. My eyes had been dry for years, and they got no worse. The summer of my treatment bloomed with clear, warm days. Some part of each was beach time for me. I was extra-careful about using sunscreen. I experienced no noticeable skin reaction and finished the summer with slightly less tan than usual. My experience does not imply that people should expect absolutely no side effects from any of the new drugs. Side effects happen, but not to everyone. And they occur with direct-acting antivirals much, much less than they did with interferon.

After week two I called Maria for a report on my viral load. "It's undetectable!" she said. I was elated. The next week it was undetectable too. The viral report after that was due just after the British Columbia Day long weekend.

Again I called Maria for the number. She said my viral count wasn't in yet because lab staff had probably been away on the Monday holiday. She said she would let me know the viral load at my next appointment.

BC Day also seemed to prolong my payment stress. The second delivery of $38,000 worth of pills was to come in less than a week. My insurance plan said it would pay for the pills directly this time, and I had taken an assignment-of-payment form directly to the insurance office. I assumed everything was A-okay. Just a day before the delivery date of the second batch of pills, I called Pacific Blue Cross.

A woman named Elizabeth answered the phone. Because of our shared name, we hit it off. She said the company was working on my claim. She looked for it and said, "It is in our building, but I can't find it." I wound up registering for an online fax service and faxing a new form to her. When I asked whether my drug bill would be paid, she said, "The Claims Department is working on it as of this moment." That was less than a day before the drugs were to be delivered. I lost sleep that night.

The next morning, still unsure whether the drugs would come because of the payment issue, I tacked the black-on-yellow signs onto my shed and a tree. By early afternoon a courier truck was rumbling down my driveway. Pacific Blue Cross had held true to its promise of a rush and paid my claim before I had to reach for plastic cards. They paid off my earlier credit card drug-spend too.

The next day, I took the ferry to Vancouver, stopping at a Starbucks on the highway in North Vancouver to take my pills with a coffee at precisely 7:30 a.m. When I arrived at the clinic, I had one big question for Maria.

I had been told after my FibroScan that my liver had measured F3 on the METAVIR fibrosis scale, which is the highest stage of fibrosis before cirrhosis. I wondered how close I was to advanced liver damage and was hoping that Maria would be able to tell me. We sat in a tiny office crammed with shelves that were crammed with thick binders labeled with the titles of clinical studies. Another nurse strode in and rummaged through the binders. "What was my actual numerical score within the F3?" I asked Maria.

The FibroScan scoring system assigns numbers from 1 to 75. A higher number indicates a greater degree of liver damage. Maria peered at the computer screen and said, "You scored 12.7. That's stage 3."

The other nurse, hovering close by because the room was so small, glanced at my chart and piped in, "No. That's cirrhosis."

"No," Maria said, "12.7 is a 3."

"Nope. Look at the graph," said her colleague. She leaned over Maria's shoulder, plunked at the computer, and pulled up a bookmarked page on a browser. Colored bars spread across a web page. The bars were somewhat blurry—the JPG file had probably been blown up. There were two shades of green bars and a yellow bar that indicated progressive densities of fibrosis. An orange bar, which was clearly marked F3, merged into an orange-red bar. Then came a red bar, and a dark red bar after that. The dark red color stretched halfway across the screen, indicating that advanced cirrhosis is as long as the other stages put together. To confuse matters further, the bars showed different starting points for each of the four fibrosis stages, depending on the type of liver disease (hep B, hep C, HIV coinfection, fatty liver disease, and others). There were a few ways to look at the chart, but my 12.7 seemed to lie right on the line between fibrosis and cirrhosis. My stomach got a car-crash feeling.

Then Maria said that my latest viral count was less than

40 (virions per milliliter of blood), but it was detectable. That was a lot lower than 176,000, but "detectable" was infinitely more than zero. I didn't want even a single nano-tiny steel-coated virus thing swimming around in my blood.

Maria noticed my dismay and reviewed some key concepts for me. "Undetectable" in hep speak means less than 15 viral bits per milliliter of blood. The PCR test cannot isolate the virus in such low amounts. The reason my virus had reappeared with a small but detectable number must have been because a tiny amount of hepatitis C RNA—too little for the test to find—had lingered in my blood. The virus would have reproduced once again and become detectable. "That happens," she said. "Don't worry. It's a tiny amount."

Back home, I worried about the tiny number of virions that remained in my blood and pulled up chart after chart that showed how FibroScan scores line up with the METAVIR fibrosis scale. Most of the charts were confusing because they color-coded and correlated many, many scores with many types of hepatitis. But one chart, courtesy of Nezam H. Afdhal of Harvard's Beth Israel Deaconess Medical Center, a teaching hospital for Harvard Medical School, seemed clear to me. It showed where the scores fall within the four stages of liver damage for hepatitis C:

less than 7.0 = fibrosis stage F0–F1
greater than 7.0 = fibrosis stage F2
greater than 9.5 = fibrosis stage F3
greater than 12.0 = fibrosis stage F4 (cirrhosis)

Oops. I was at 12.7.

## July 1969, Next Day

# SHOTS

AS THAT MORNING grew hot, my friends and I continued to stand by the edge of Route 40, thrusting our thumbs at occasional cars speeding by. I hardly ever sweat, but my T-shirt felt like a soggy dishrag. We had been thumbing for hours. Cactus-spotted desert spread out flat on each side of the road. There had been a long gap after the last few cars passed by. Traffic would pick up in an hour or two, I reasoned, when people were heading places for lunch. The four of us shared an early lunch: a bag of Fritos from my baby pack and the last of our water. I still had a few cans of milk for Della, but that wouldn't last.

Finally, an El Camino, a truck–car hybrid that was popular in the '60s, sped toward us, blowing up dust. The truck passed us and our outstretched thumbs but in a second it slowed and backed up. As it rolled to a stop, I saw two men and two women squeezed into its three-person cab. Judging from the long hair on all of them and the beards on the men, I figured they were hippies. Ryan and Peter must have thought so too because they smiled and nodded at me.

"Where to?" asked the driver, the burlier of the two burly men.

"Santa Fe," Peter said.

"Same as us." The driver said, motioning toward the vehicle's open back. "Get in."

I threw my bag into the back, boosted Della over the rail, and climbed in with Peter and Ryan. I sat in the passenger-side corner next to the cab, using the half-full duffel as a lumpy pillow. My daughter squatted on my lap. It was easy to hear the chatter in the cab through a three-inch gap in the window panels. I heard about the Harley one of the men was going to pick up somewhere and of an encounter with "pigs" that the passenger-side man claimed one of the women had mishandled. The scraggly-haired blond woman protested, and then the man, who was seated between the two women, slapped her. "Shut yer fuckin' mouth," he said.

These were not hippies; they were bikers. I could see Ryan and Peter had come to the same conclusion. One after the other, my traveling partners frowned and shook their heads slightly. I faced away from the cab, trying to be invisible. The bikers were getting louder, arguing. Peter, Ryan, and I scrunched closer together on the truck bed.

"As soon as they stop anywhere, we'll get out, thank them, and say good-bye," Peter whispered to me. "We'll find another ride."

"We told them we were going to Santa Fe," Ryan said.

"We'll say we changed our plans," said Peter. "We were planning to go all the way to Taos, right?"

"That doesn't make sense. Taos is *after* Santa Fe," I said. "Let's tell them about my pay. We can say we think we should turn around and go to the Western Union in Kingman. That's the opposite way from where they're going. The closer we are to the truth, the easier it will be to convince them."

"What if they follow us so they can rip off the money order?" Peter asked.

"Why don't we say our friends Teena and Raccoon are there and we're going to ask them to lend us money?" I suggested. "That's not as easy a rip-off."

Peter and Ryan nodded.

So we had a plan. But plans go awry. What occurred later that day in the desert was another possible cause of my infection with hepatitis C.

As the El Camino sped along the highway in searing July heat, Della snuggled against me. Ryan and Peter braced themselves against the opposite rail. I listened to jabber coming from the cab and gradually figured out the bikers' names. There were Eddie, the bearded, meaty driver, and Squatch, his bearded, bulb-nosed sidekick. Letty, a platinum blond with sunken cheeks and dark roots growing an inch above her scalp, sat next to the driver. The woman with the greasy, stringy, yellow-blond hair was Babs.

Squatch and Letty must have heard me talking with the guys, and they turned their heads. The conversation in the back of the truck ended. Squatch pushed the window panels so that they were fully open on the passenger side in front of me. "Pass that over here, will yuh?"

He motioned toward the twenty-four-pack of beer in the middle of the truck bed. Ryan hoisted it through the window opening. The truck swerved as Letty pressed against Eddie while Squatch swung the cans onto the floor. The bikers closed the window. Soon they were all guzzling beer, including the driver.

Minutes passed with quiet among both groups in the El Camino. Babs tossed a beer can out the window and cracked open another. She leaned out of the open side window just a foot from where I was seated and held out the can to me. "Want some?" she asked.

"No thanks."

"Ah, come on. We're partying."

I didn't know how to respond, but Squatch ended the conversation by lunging over Babs. He grabbed the can from her hand. "Enough for you! You don't git to party after yapping off to the pigs." He held a can of beer in each hand. He slurped down his own, threw the can past Babs's head and out the window, and started drinking from the other can. Babs slumped toward the door.

The car suddenly turned left onto a narrower highway. This wasn't the route to Santa Fe. Ryan, Peter, and I glanced at each other.

Squatch opened the window. "Detour," he said. "Gonna get some grub."

We stared at each other, relieved. This would be the stop where we could make our excuses and say good-bye to our chauffeurs. After what seemed like forever we came to a sign welcoming us to the Grand Canyon. The truck rolled to a stop.

Eddie got out of the driver's side, walked to the back, and said, "Lunchtime. Get movin'."

We shuffled into the restaurant at the Grand Canyon National Park, and Eddie directed us to a booth behind the bikers. "Don't go nowhere," he said.

"The bathroom?" I asked.

"One atta time."

Peter, Ryan, and I (with Della) took turns visiting the washrooms. As I combed wind tangles from my hair, I thought about pictures I had seen of the canyon. We would walk outside and view the majestic gorge and tell the bikers we wanted to meet our friends in Kingman. It was in the opposite direction from their route, so they would leave us at the restaurant. We would catch another ride with someone else. We would be a lot more careful about the car we chose.

As I slipped past Peter to get into the booth, I whispered, "Can we get away from them?"

He nodded. I glanced at the bikers, and as they returned my gaze I did my best to smile graciously. Their table was full of plates of ketchupy fries and cans of beer.

My group finished our cheeseburgers and dug through our pockets to pay the bill, and the bikers motioned for us to follow them outside. Carrying Della, I tried to peer over the fence to see the canyon, but the fence was too high. Eddie said, "Back in the truck. Time to go."

"Thanks but we're thinking we should turn around and go back to Kingman to meet our friends," Peter said. "We're going to ask them to loan us the bus fare to Taos. We're planning to take the bus to Taos."

Ryan went to lift our bag from the truck box, but Eddie said, "Not so fast."

Ryan stopped. Peter and I froze.

"Yeah, don't worry yerself, yer comin' with us," Eddie said. "We're warring with the citizens, but youze is righteous folk. We're takin' ya all the way to Taos. Git in the truck."

We climbed into the back.

Eddie and Squatch stood outside of the El Camino and debated which road to take. They drank more beer. Inside the cab Letty and Babs drank beer. I thought we would just go back the way we came and onto the main highway, so the discussion of driving routes didn't make sense. Maybe the bikers knew a shortcut to Taos, I reasoned. Soon we were rolling along on whatever route they had decided to take.

All four bikers continued their beer drinking, and then Squatch pulled out a bottle of something brown from behind the seat. He passed it to Eddie, who passed it to Letty, who tried to pass it over Squatch to Babs. Babs put out her hand but Squatch grabbed the bottle. "You were too fuckin' plastered when we got stopped," he said.

"Aw, come on, Squatchie."

"Okay. Head back. Open up." He poured liquor down her throat until she began to choke.

"Enough. She'll git her punishment," Eddie said.

Squatch stopped pouring. Babs coughed and choked.

The bikers were quiet again, and after a while Babs fumbled with something below the seat and my line of vision. Then she flung her arm out the window. There was a ribbon tied below her bicep. With stringlike hair whipping around her face, leaning out the window in the breeze, she jabbed a needle into the crook of her arm. She sank against the door, closed her eyes, and stayed silent. The truck sped along.

After a while the ride turned rough. The truck bumped and shuddered. We had left the highway and turned into a rough dirt road. No other vehicles were in sight. The desert spread out dry and bleak. Few cacti grew here. Boulders and angular rocks spotted the otherwise flat ground. It looked like a different planet, unfit for human life. The road widened and then ended, and the truck groaned to a stop. The bikers got out.

"Coffee break," Squatch called. There was no coffee. We all got out, except for Della, who was napping on the blanket in the back of the truck.

Eddie pushed Babs in front of him. "Time for your punishment. Git out there." The biker men guzzled beer. Eddie drained his can and tossed it at Babs, and she caught it. Her other hand held a smoking cigarette. It swayed with her body as she took a drag.

"Out there!" Eddie said, pointing.

Babs crushed the cigarette and trotted into the dusty flatland holding the beer can. Squatch rummaged inside the truck, behind the seat. He came out with a bottle of whiskey and a rifle. He took a swing of the brew and gave Eddie the rifle.

Eddie grabbed the bottle too and gulped some down.

Babs turned toward the men, her lips pursed and snarky looking. "Here?" she asked.

"Keep goin'," Eddie told her. "She's gittin' her punishment," he announced to us as we stood by the side of the truck.

Babs trotted into the dusty desert. When she was about thirty yards out, she turned around. "Here?"

Eddie turned to Squatch. "Wha'dya think?"

"A bit short."

"Keep goin'," Eddie said.

Babs continued another ten yards, turned, and stopped.

"Good enough, I'd guess," Squatch said.

"Sure," Eddie said. He took another swig of whiskey. He placed the bottle on the ground and cocked the rifle.

Babs plunked the beer can on top of her head. She tottered and it fell. She picked it up and tried again. She moved the can to different spots on her head. Finally it rested on her cranium. She appeared defiant. The can teetered, but it held.

Eddie stood with his feet seemingly glued to their position. Above the knees, he was swaying. "Check this out," he said to us.

Babs swayed more than Eddie.

Eddie held the rifle to his shoulder and squinted into the sight. He tottered, steadied himself, and wobbled again. Then he pulled the trigger. My ears felt like they were caving in from thunder. A sharp scent of gunpowder permeated the air, and gray-black smoke wisped from the gun barrel. Eddie had shot at Babs. It was a long few seconds before I could force myself to look to where she had been standing.

*CHAPTER 10*

# ANOTHER
# LETTER

T HE REMAINING WEEKS of treatment comprised daily
pill-taking, viral load counts each week, blood panels
every second week, and a call to Maria five days after
each viral load test to hear the results. I took the ferry to
the GI clinic the day after my third cooler of pills arrived,
and I visited my general practitioner, Dr. Radev, once. As
for the weekly viral load tests, I tested clear after that single
detectable blip, and after that, and after that. I downed the
last two pills on October 8, 2014. Two days later my treatment became obsolete.

The Food and Drug Administration approved Harvoni
on October 10, 2014. A week later Health Canada approved
it. The drug was the first one-tablet, once-a-day regimen
that eliminated the need for interferon. Harvoni combines
Sovaldi and ledipasvir, both from Gilead. The drug's success rate in clinical trials varied between 94 and 99 percent

sustained virologic response for a twelve-week treatment. In Canada, instead of paying a total of $115,000 for two pills each day, genotype 1b patients like me could now pay $84,000 for the newest, easiest miracle cure. (In the U.S., patients with genotype 1b had paid $150,000 for the two pills a day and would now pay $94,500 for the new treatment.) Those with genotype 1a could also take Harvoni. After further trials, in November 2015 the FDA approved Harvoni for genotypes 4, 5, and 6. Most people with hep C opted for Harvoni, and Gilead's profits climbed.

As the drug company shareholders were cheering, employees with health plans were losing out. Toward the end of my treatment, most plans had yet to obtain a discount on the new direct-acting antivirals. I got my drugs early and slipped through the cracks. But soon insurance companies were refusing to pay for the drugs without a huge increase in premiums. Employers generally chose less of a plan over more of a premium. The nurses' union in my province had just announced that its extended medical plan through Pacific Blue Cross was moving to Fair PharmaCare. Hep C drugs, including Sovaldi, Galexos, Harvoni, and the emerging AbbVie combination Holkira Pak (Viekira Pak in the U.S.), were not on the PharmaCare list. Therefore, the nurses' plan would refuse to pay for the new direct-acting antivirals for nurses who had hepatitis C, nurse Emily Doyle explained to me. "It's a terrible thing," she commented about the lack of coverage.

I was talking with her as I rolled up my shirt sleeve, preparing for a final hep B vaccination. "I probably don't need this," I said as Emily pulled the plunger on a hypodermic full of pale yellow fluid. It was early December. That morning I had finished marking the last of my courses, had twice gone for walks with neighbors, and had received an early Christmas email greeting from a friend who was traveling to Mexico. Although I was yet to get my twelve-week viral load results, I was feeling optimistic.

"I think I've cleared the hep," I added.

"That's wonderful," Emily remarked, jabbing the needle into my arm. As she packed the used hypodermic for disposal, I was surprised she didn't ask about my treatment, like all the other shot-giving or blood-taking people I had met since the early summer had done. They had each asked the question with concerned demeanors that communicated that they were sorry I had to endure heavy side effects. They had all assumed I had been using interferon. Each time I had set them straight. By this time, though, news of non-interferon direct-acting antivirals had spread through the health care professions. Emily listened as I explained that I had completed twelve weeks of direct-acting antivirals with virtually no side effects.

"I've heard about something like that," she said, a big smile spreading across her pretty face. She turned toward the computer and brought up a web page that announced the approval of Harvoni.

About a week later I talked about Harvoni with my musician friend Adam Bailey. He said he was getting more and more anxious about being treated, and now his doctor had proposed the new drug.

"But I'd have to pay for it." He said he couldn't afford the price, so he was still considering the older regimen with interferon (his genotype was 1a, so the combo I had taken wasn't an option). In addition to being a musician, Adam works as a home automation technician installing automatic lighting, thermostats, and other high-tech comfort gadgets. His hep remained symptomless, so he was working steadily all over the Sea-to-Sky Corridor, the mountainous area between Vancouver and Whistler. He was insured under his wife's plan, which initially wouldn't pay for his treatment with direct-acting antivirals. Ironically, his wife worked as a claims adjuster for a health insurance company.

"How do you take this interferon?" Adam asked.

I explained it had to be injected into fatty tissues. I said a friend had received the injections in his back.

"You can imagine forty-eight weeks of that!" Adam said, aghast.

On top of that, his doctor still wanted do a biopsy. Adam said he couldn't help being squeamish. "I just don't like thinking about it," he said.

I reminded him that my doctor did FibroScans instead of biopsies. I suggested he call Dr. Ramji, and he did. Adam's appointment was the week before Christmas. I told Adam I hoped to see him at a New Year's Eve party, but he didn't show up.

A week after New Year's, which was the date I retired as a university instructor, Maria said I had achieved what some people had begun to call a twelve-week SVR. In the old lingo a clear, twelve-week viral count would have been considered just an EVR (early virologic response). Sustained virologic response would be declared only when six months had elapsed after treatment. Dr. Ramji assured me that with the new drugs, a twelve-week count would be a strong indication the hep C was gone. Maria, though, was used to managing clinical trials that demanded long-term statistics. She insisted I wait longer before she would confirm an all-clear. Relapse—the return of the hepatitis C virus after a time of dormancy—had occurred after EVR in one-third of patients who had taken interferon. I hadn't used it, but my treatment was still very new, Maria reminded me. Nonetheless, I had followed directions to the proverbial T and had received a string of undetectable viral loads. I told myself I had to be on the upper end of success rates for a cure.

During the first week of spring 2015, I stood at the counter at LifeLabs. A young woman with brown, crinkly hair tied back from her face took my requisition sheet. I asked to lie down, and she led me to a bed in the examining room. This would probably be the last blood test I'd need for many months. I was 98 percent sure I had cleared the hep. Maria had said in order to be 100 percent sure, I should wait twice as long—twenty-four weeks—to get a final test. This was that test.

Jody, the lab technician, chatted amiably with me while I lay on the cot. As she tied a latex tourniquet around my arm, I clamped my eyes shut so that I wouldn't see the needle. I asked Jody whether she thought the number of hepatitis C patients had been declining since Harvoni came on the market. She said she saw a lot of hep C patients but couldn't tell where the numbers were going because she had barely started her career. She jabbed the needle into the crook of my arm. It hurt.

A week later my 98 percent estimate of a cure pushed me into dark thoughts about the 2 percent possibility. They woke me at four in the morning. I recalled the time I had entered a draw in a supermarket in Florida. It was a singles' night, and about two hundred men and women roamed the store. They plunked groceries into their carts and gravitated toward whomever they thought was cute in the produce or bakery aisle. They also each dropped a ticket into the draw box. At the end of the night, while some shoppers walked away with a date, I left the store with a microwave oven. My name had been drawn out of two hundred draw tickets. That was four times as unlikely an event as a hepatitis relapse, at least according to the odds I had projected. I reminded myself that Dr. Ramji had predicted only a seventeen out of twenty chance of a cure. I had heard many stories about relapses after the old treatments, and there was no telling what would happen with the new ones. My 98 percent estimate must be a delusion, I thought.

A few hours later the sun hit my eyes and I gave up trying to sleep. I stumbled from my bedroom into the dining room. I skipped breakfast and tried to read the news, but I couldn't concentrate. At 8:30 a.m., when Maria usually arrived at the GI clinic, when I knew I should call, I avoided the irreversible step of calling her. Judging from the series of nondetectable viral counts since early in my treatment, I recalculated my chances of being clear of the virus. I was 99 percent sure I was okay. Yet I was shaky. If you were on an airplane and the pilot said there's trouble, but don't worry, there's only a 1 percent chance of a crash, you'd scream, cry, or cling to your loved one, certain the end is coming.

I stared at the phone, trying to convince myself I should call Maria to find out if I had achieved a twenty-four-week sustained virologic response. Meanwhile, my husband plunked away at his computer on the dining table, preaching to me about programmatic software, an automatic system for buying online advertising. Al is a media buyer, and he likes to talk about his job. Usually I'm happy to listen, but his words seemed to fade into the background like Muzak. My mind was focused elsewhere. The plane was going to crash, I believed, even though that was improbable.

I thought about my niece Sandy. I hoped she would be cured. My west coast family all knew about my illness, but Sandy and her mother, Mary, were the only members of my larger number of east coast relations who knew I had hep C. Your family can be your biggest support when you're stricken with the demon—but not all of them may have that capacity. Soon after my diagnosis, I learned that if I were to reveal my disease to anyone, including my family, I should consider the person's sensitivities and prejudices before deciding whether to tell them I had hep and put aside ample time to talk with the person so that I could explain the background of my disease.

My long-distance family lived three thousand miles away, so for the year following my diagnosis, I chose to tell only Mary about my illness. She seemed to be the most sympathetic long-distance listener of the bunch. Of course Sandy, her daughter, was sympathetic too because she also had hep. I continued staring at the phone and considered calling Mary, who might help me muster the courage to call Maria.

"Are you making a call?" Al asked.

"No, I'm making coffee." The coffee maker stood next to the phone. So I made a pot of coffee and poured a cup for Al. I poured a cup for myself and grabbed one of the mini cinnamon buns I had bought at Costco. I decided to relax on the sofa with a novel and call the nurse at exactly 10 a.m. That was twenty-two minutes away. I couldn't relax. I couldn't follow the storyline. I checked my watch every two minutes as 10 a.m. approached. When three zeroes appeared on the digital readout, I forced myself to get up and make the call. I got Maria's voice mail and left a message asking her to call me when she had time.

I don't know how I got through the next three hours. Al sensed what was happening and kept asking me to call. At 12:55 p.m. he punched Maria's number into his cell and handed the phone to me.

"It's undetectable! I *knew* the virus would be gone," Maria said. "That's what's happening these days."

AFTER YOU'RE CURED, the beans are easier to spill. My hep C had cleared, and I felt a buzz of new energy.

I called my youngest sister, Irene, to talk about my mother, who was spry for a near-centenarian but weighed eighty pounds and looked like a famished human Tweety Bird. We discussed my mother's housing situation. She had the option of moving five hours north to Ocala, Florida, where both Irene and Mary owned homes. Both houses would be better situations for my mother, but I preferred Mary's.

Irene asked why, when I visited Ocala, I had stayed at Mary's instead of with her.

"Mary has an Internet connection, which I need for my work," I said.

"I have an Internet connection," Irene said.

"Mary has some nice roads around her house, and I like to go for walks to keep healthy."

"I have very nice roads around my house where you can walk."

"Well, I like staying in the room Mary has with the connecting bathroom."

That's where our niece Sandy stays, my sister declared. "She has hepatitis C, and it sits there for two weeks in bathrooms. It can sit on something for seven to ten days."

I had never told Irene I had hep, because she lived with my mother, and Irene was a gossip. I didn't want my elderly mother to worry about me. But it never occurred to me that anyone in my family would propagate a stigma that is so hurtful to people who have hep. So I spewed out my story to Irene. I told her I had contracted hepatitis C from a blood transfusion after my daughter was born. I told Irene she was wrong, wrong, wrong. It is impossible to get hep from a bathroom. It can be transmitted only with blood-to-blood contact.

She said she had done her own research and was sure it could happen.

"I'm writing a book on the topic," I said. "I've read hundreds of research studies. It's impossible for that to happen!"

"But, but..."

I hung up.

IT WAS MANY weeks before I talked with Irene again. During that time, I poured out my sister's story to Anahid Aslanyan, who understood my distress. I had met Anahid through Shirley Barger, the retiree who had been a UNIX administrator at the City College of San Francisco. Anahid had been attending Shirley's support group for people infected with hepatitis C.

Anahid lives with her husband in Potrero Hill, about a ten-minute drive from downtown San Francisco. She spends a lot of time painting. When she's not doing that you will probably find her cuddling her black dog, Shadow, a fourteen-pound Chihuahua-dachshund cross. As I talked with Anahid, Shadow dragged a blanket along the floor and wiggled under it. "He's the best dog in the world. He's so sweet," Anahid said in a cheery Armenian accent. "You know, I've never had children. I'd never experienced this kind of love. I can't wait in the morning to just love him and kiss him."

Anahid graduated from the San Francisco Art Institute in the 1980s and has shown her paintings and whimsical mixed-media pieces in the U.S., Armenia, and the Czech Republic. Her work blends nature scenes with a gentle touch of surrealism. The colors are vibrant but not overwhelming. It's the kind of art I like to hang on my walls.

The demon entered her body in 1974, when she was in her early twenties. Anahid had been using a Dalkon Shield, an intrauterine device, to avoid pregnancy, and she started having a lot of pain. She attributed it to the shield. In the 1980s the largest tort (wrongful act) lawsuit in history was filed against the A.H. Robins Company, the maker of the horseshoe-crab-shaped IUD, and the company went bankrupt. At least 200,000 claimants suffered infections, perforations of the uterus, hysterectomies, miscarriages, or ectopic pregnancies because of the device, and seventeen women died, according to authors Anna Bahr and Kathleen Byrne, who each wrote a story about the debacle.

Anahid's pain became unbearable. Her mother took her to a hospital, where a doctor gave her antibiotics and told her mother Anahid had gonorrhea. After a week, the doctor said it was time for Anahid go home. "But I yelled and screamed so bad," Anahid told me. "I saved my own life by yelling and screaming." After agreeing to do further tests, the doctor inserted a needle through her vagina and found blood in her abdomen; her fallopian tube had burst from an ectopic pregnancy, which had started in her tube because the IUD had shielded her uterus. In surgery, as the medical team removed the embryo and repaired the tube, she lost a lot of blood. She said the doctors replaced it with hep-tainted blood.

Like many people with hepatitis C, over the years Anahid had experienced vague physical problems. One time, when her art was being exhibited in a group show, the gallery offered free drinks to the artists. Somebody gave her a strong vodka cranberry cocktail, which set off pelvic inflammation for months. She didn't know she had hep C, but she knew something was wrong. She began to avoid alcohol. "My doctor said, 'This has nothing to do with alcohol,' but I knew it did," she said. "After I was diagnosed it made sense. Something was there. There was a scar, adhesions. That's what set off the inflammation." Ever since, she has averaged a glass of wine or a margarita a year.

Then, in 2008, an old friend from college was in the hospital with liver cancer. The woman had injected drugs for many years. She had cleaned up, but not before she contracted hepatitis C. Anahid knew her friend had hep, but the woman wouldn't talk about it and never sought treatment. She kept her symptoms from her own doctors. After a while it was too late to save her liver. Anahid visited her in the hospital. "She looked like a horror movie," Anahid said, adding that she felt anger toward her friend because she had neglected her health. But mostly Anahid was sad.

One day Anahid felt a heavy pain in her back. She thought it was from the stress of her friend's condition. She asked her doctor for some tests. "I had to twist her arm, and then she gave me a blood test," Anahid said. It revealed abnormally high liver enzymes. The doctor sent her for a CT scan, which combines X rays taken at different angles to create detailed images of body tissues. The images showed liver scarring. Other tests revealed that she had a viral load of just under 3 million with genotype 1a hepatitis C.

While Anahid was going through the tests, her friend died.

Anahid couldn't stop thinking about her friend, except when she was thinking about the virus that was attacking her. She believed hep C was a death sentence. Her mind spun down an ever-descending spiral. She went on anti-depressants, but within a year she stopped. She crashed. Then the depression lifted and life became as normal as she could make it.

In 2011, a gastroenterologist at the California Pacific Medical Center (Sutter Health) performed a biopsy. It showed that her liver was close to cirrhosis. Anahid asked to be treated, but those were interferon days. The doctor said she shouldn't take the drug because she had already been depressed. He said new drugs were being developed that would be far easier on her mind and body. She agreed with him and began a wait for direct-acting antivirals.

She started reading the HCV Advocate, the newsletter of San Francisco's hepatitis C community, where she learned about clinical trials and the new medicines. "I used to read it out and underline everything. I was waiting, waiting, waiting for something to come out before it got really bad and I had complications." Some of the things she learned were scary. She heard about people whose portal vein or capillaries had burst. The portal vein carries blood from the gastrointestinal tract to the heart, by way of the liver, and cirrhosis can block its flow. Anahid joined Shirley's support group and began taking milk thistle, turmeric, and other liver remedies. She loves nature and often went on hikes. "Of course that's not going to get rid of your virus," she said, "but it helps."

"It was a hopeless situation for many years," she recalled, "waiting for the drugs to come out."

My niece Sandy had the same problem as Anahid. They had been depressed, so they couldn't be treated for their hepatitis C with the old interferon-based treatments. When Harvoni entered the medical consciousness during the 2014–15 winter holidays, Sandy's doctor said he was willing to prescribe it because it didn't cause depression. Sandy applied to her insurer to cover the drug. "She's going to be up against the money problem if the insurance company says no," my sister Mary said. "The doctor told me that if you're not close to dying they won't pay for the medication."

The insurer, Prestige Health Choice, asked that Sandy have her liver tested. Mary was daunted by the invasiveness of a biopsy and asked that Sandy get a FibroScan. The company insisted on a biopsy. The doctor explained to my sister that Sandy would have a CT scan, then a needle would be inserted into her liver, then there would be another CT scan. The biopsy had to be done, as it could be the deciding factor for the insurance company. Mary waited as Sandy lay in the procedure room. "I'm outside of the door ready to collapse," Mary said. "It's not a nice thing, that liver biopsy."

The biopsy showed Sandy's liver damage as stage 2. Prestige Health Choice refused to pay for the $95,000 drug, stating, "Your request does not meet pharmacy coverage guidelines. Patient does not have Stage 3 or Stage 4 hepatic fibrosis."[1]

In late summer of 2015, Mary continued to agonize about her daughter's hep C. Sandy couldn't work and Mary couldn't afford the high-priced pills. Sandy sent an appeal letter to the company:

> My Mother helped me write this appeal letter. She is better able to communicate my feelings toward this insidious disease, hepatitis C.
>
> I also suffer from schizophrenia. This disease carries a stigma. Most people in the community do not understand that schizophrenia is a chemical imbalance that could affect anyone, even themselves. It's just the luck of the draw whether you have it. People also don't understand that schizophrenia can be treated. I am being treated. My meds keep the disease at bay and keep me stable. I take my meds on schedule and am trying to lead as normal a life as possible.
>
> Unfortunately, I have more to deal with than schizophrenia as I also have hepatitis C. This disease, which can eventually kill me, also carries a stigma. People don't

understand that it's impossible to contract hep C just from being around me. But I don't hide my disease from them. There are some casual routes to infection and I am obligated to tell people I have hep C. When I tell some people this they back away from me as if I had Ebola. Attempting to get any type of menial employment is out of the question as soon as I mention hepatitis C.

This kind of stigma is hard to face on top of the burden of schizophrenia. I am trying very hard to be a productive member of the community. The disease I cannot ever completely conquer, schizophrenia, is being made worse by a disease that's completely curable, hepatitis C. I am told that Harvoni cures 100% of people with very few side effects.

Meanwhile, hepatitis C has side effects that go beyond liver damage and I'm sure I'm suffering from some of them. When I have bouts of depression, knowing I have hepatitis C in my body makes me more depressed. When I am depressed I can sometimes forget to take my meds for schizophrenia, which is the last thing I want to do. If I forget to take my meds I can start hallucinating. Then everything I've done to try to be a good person becomes a shambles. Getting treatment for hepatitis C is actually also a schizophrenia treatment for me. It shouldn't matter what stage of hepatitis C I have because the disease is making another extremely serious illness, worse. As such, I am more vulnerable than most patients and would be considered sicker than most patients I know. I desperately need the treatment for Hep C with Harvoni. Please help me.

# ROCKS

THE GUNSHOT NOISE receded. I blinked at the smoke and gazed into the barren landscape. There was Babs, still standing. She lurched but didn't fall. I had thought I'd see death, but she was alive.

Eddie had shot the beer can off her head. I felt as if I were waking from a bad dream into a morning that itself seemed like a dream but could be real. I was in awe that Babs stood there without a scratch. She smirked as she took a cigarette from her pocket. But the nightmare continued.

Squatch nudged Letty toward the truck. She bent into the cab and picked up four empty beer cans. She ran up to Babs, plunked the cans on the gravel beside her, and scampered back to Squatch. Babs lit the cigarette and positioned a beer can on her head. Eddie reloaded and cocked the rifle. Once again he shot the can off of Bab's head. The cigarette hung from her mouth. She wavered but didn't flinch. Eddie repeated the show three more times. Each can kaboomed, flew up for a long second, and clattered to the dusty ground. The smell of gunpowder coated everything. I froze throughout the volley, feeling as if the world were spinning around me but I was somewhere else, possibly in the Phantom Zone, observing and getting ready to see a murder.

But Eddie never missed a can. When the smoke from the last can cleared, Babs took a few drags from her cigarette and started walking toward us.

"Not so fast," Eddie hollered. "Turn sideways."

She stopped and turned her side to her observers. Her wobbly stance became more obvious. She was slim and swaying, like a twig in the wind.

"Do it," Eddie shouted.

Babs clenched the cigarette in her mouth. It had burned half-way down. Eddie raised the rifle. It boomed.

"Owww," Babs yelped. "Eddie, you burned me," she said, wiping soot from her lip.

"Well, ya gotta stand still. Let's go again."

"You blew it apart," she said, holding the cigarette outward and showing a distorted stub of a filter.

"Okay. Enough for now," Eddie said. He held out the rifle and turned to Peter. He motioned toward me. "Wanna try it with her?"

Peter, whom I had learned I couldn't always trust, did the one best thing he had ever done for me. His words remain etched in my mind. He said, "Na. She's been good lately."

We all headed back to the El Camino. As the bikers were getting into the front, Eddie said to Babs, "Ya didn't finish yer punishment. I'm tired. You drive." He handed her the keys. Babs turned the truck onto the road going to the highway but didn't get that far.

She was stoned on whatever she had put into her arm and she was drunk as well. Her foot smashed hard into the accelerator. The truck whipped around the dead end and screeched over rock-strewn road. The vehicle plunged ahead, teetering with its right wheels slipping in and out of a gully. The truck hit a boulder and flipped. My friends and I shot out of the back.

I landed hard on hot rocks under 115-degree sun. My head smashed onto rocks. My back smashed onto rocks. Heat bit into my back where the rocks had ripped through my shirt. Blood puddled around my head. The scene swirled into nothing. I don't know how long it took for me to come to, but when I did, I saw Della standing over me. I remember intense physical pain, pain so bad that I wished I'd die to get rid of it. But worse than that was the anguish over my daughter. She was crying and covered with blood. *Oh God,* I thought, even though my own clear-light religion had no god. *Make my daughter okay. Make her safe.*

It took at least an hour for an ambulance to come. I was surprised it came at all—we were so far from everything. Eventually I learned that a rancher had spotted us. I also learned that my daughter didn't have even the tiniest abrasion. The blood on her clothes was mine, not hers. I had hit the rocks with my head and back. She had fallen on my stomach, which cushioned her.

Peter was fine as well. In the army he had learned to jump from a plane, and when he was tossed from the truck, he vaulted like a paratrooper and landed on his feet. He took care of Della until I was out of the hospital.

The bikers were badly injured. A nurse told me one of the women—I don't know which—had suffered brain damage. One of the bikers fractured both of his legs in many places. Ryan broke his back, spent the summer in the same room as that biker, and when he was released from hospital, he became a biker too.

After the ambulance had pulled up to the hospital near Flagstaff, I was unconscious for a while. I woke under glaring lights, lying on my stomach as doctors cleaned out gravel from the crisscross of lacerations on my back. A nurse shaved the back of my head and swabbed up blood. "I'm giving you something for the pain," she said. She plunged a syringe into a cannula taped to my hand. My mind clouded over with whatever she had given me, and through my hazy vision it seemed that the tube that ran to my hand was turning red.

When I woke again I was told I had close to fifty stitches in my head, sprained vertebrae, and extensive cuts and bruises on my back. But I was never sure what had happened in the operating room. After sending a request for records to the main Flagstaff hospital (I'm not sure which of eight area hospitals I was in), I never got anything back. But I believe that I may have had a blood transfusion. Doctors had prepared three units of blood for me after my postpartum hemorrhage, but according to the American Red Cross, in traumatic car accidents, up to 100 pints of blood can be used. If I had received a second transfusion in Arizona, there may have been a greater chance that it gave me hepatitis C.

During the next few days in the Flagstaff hospital, my mind remained fuzzy from Demerol and from pain, which the Demerol didn't kill. On the fourth morning, a nurse wheeled me to the end of a long hall and into an office where Peter sat arguing with an administrator. She glared at him through slitty eyes and asked him to pay about $2,500 U.S. for my surgery and inpatient care, which would be close to $17,000 now.

"We don't have that kind of money," Peter said.

"We don' have the money," I slurred, parroting him though my pain-muddled mind.

"You could mortgage your house," she said.

"We don't have a house," Peter said.

"You could get a loan through your bank," she said.

"We don't have a bank," Peter said.

"You have to pay your bill."

"We can't pay the bill."

This went on for at least an hour, maybe two. Then the woman shrugged her shoulders, leafed through a binder on her desk, and pointed a finger at a page. "We have a law in Arizona that if you can't pay your hospital bill, you don't have to pay."

"So we don' have to pay?" I slurred.

"No. You can leave now," she said.

And that was that. Peter wheeled me to the entrance, where a taxi waited. It took us to a shabby motel. Unsteady on my feet, I got out of the cab. The smiling proprietor of the motel was holding Della and handed her to me. She was a small child, probably twenty pounds, but I couldn't lift her. When I tried, I keeled over in pain.

We headed to Santa Fe and caught up with Teena and Raccoon. They stood in the bus station waving and jumping up and down when they saw us. They were both short and looked like kids. They said they had waited every day for us and were almost ready to give up. They hadn't found an accepting commune, but Raccoon's dad had sent him cash. Teena flew back to New York. The rest of us flew to Chicago, where we stayed at Raccoon's father's house. Peter, Della, and I made a little home in the basement, which I never left while I healed. It took another two months before I could carry my daughter for fifteen seconds and before my scar-riddled scalp regrew enough hair to be presentable in public. I was feeling better. Then one day, when Peter was having a hard time finding odd jobs that wouldn't check his army status, I read a newspaper article about thousands of U.S. draft dodgers and deserters who had fled to Canada.

"My dad's Canadian," I said. "His parents live in Windsor. I'm entitled to citizenship. Let's go there."

So we went. So we became soapstone carvers and later jewelers, specializing in manufacturing silver rings with cabochon stones. So I found myself in Montreal having a baby, and hemorrhaging and getting a blood transfusion that may have led to hepatitis C. Or maybe it was an earlier transfusion in Flagstaff, Arizona, that drew in the demon. Or maybe it was the razor cuts, though that possibility seems remote. Maybe it was from sex with Peter, who I believe had been injecting cocaine at least a year before we split up and who had raped me roughly and bruised me, although that is also remote.

But in the magnanimous and caring universe where the hippie yin and yang of clear light and the void or the more common notion of a god may exist, it doesn't matter how I contracted hepatitis C. It doesn't matter how all the wonderful people I met who had contracted hepatitis C had come down with their disease either. No matter what caused their infection, it's always an accident. Even though most transmissions when I was infected were through medical means, and though most later transmissions were through IV drugs, there is always uncertainty about the viral path into the body. What matters is that the disease be eradicated. And it can be. Miracle drugs can do that today, but no doctor will give you the drugs before you've been tested. As 2017 began, at least 100 million people were infected with hepatitis C, and most of them didn't know they had it. They need to be tested. That may be getting easier.

*CHAPTER 11*

# THE SWAB

I N EARLY 2015, John Lavette, the San Franciscan who led the seventy-two-person free-love entourage, also worried about paying for hepatitis C drugs. His wife, a property assessor, had a Blue Shield medical plan, but John wasn't sure it would pay for the new direct-acting antivirals. His hepatologist had just recommended he get treated with them. "He told me, as far as he's concerned, 'I'd better get this thing done now,'" John said.

John had tried and failed interferon treatment. Next he tried an early antiviral, telaprevir. That didn't work either. John, in his late sixties, was at the age when hepatitis tends to hit hardest. That's not necessarily because of physical effects; it's because liver damage advances more rapidly as people age. "It's become a matter of time," John said. "Over a long time nothing happens, and suddenly it can go into cirrhosis." His doctor suggested Harvoni, and John was anxious to move toward a cure. John had contacted a specialty pharmacist, who was helping him apply for payment assistance. "If they [the insurance company] turn me down, we're going to submit again," he said. "If that doesn't work, we're gonna go after the Gilead thing and try to work something out." The "Gilead thing" he was referring to was the company's patient support program. "They're miracle workers [the pharmacists], really. They seem to come up with a whole lot of angles."

A few weeks later, he received approval for Harvoni, the one-pill-a-day treatment that was curing almost everyone who had contracted hepatitis C. Some people were prescribed the drug for only eight weeks.

The transition from the standard treatment for hepatitis C, a year-long, hideous ordeal, to a short, easy remedy took half a year. From July through October 2014, I was treated with the breakthrough duo of Sovaldi and Galexos, the first set of hep C drugs to forgo interferon. By the beginning of 2015, interferon was mostly history in the Western world, and most patients in North America infected with the dominant genotype were being prescribed Harvoni. Patients now swallowed only one pill a day. Harvoni was the brainchild of Gilead, maker of Sovaldi and of fortunes for its shareholders. Other non-interferon drugs had entered the treatment list for particular genotypes.

The 2014 revolution of non-interferon hep C treatments had made the prognosis much better for millions of people still infected with HCV, but among those who had been diagnosed, many had to wait months or years for treatment. In the United States most health plans would pay the exorbitant cost of the drugs only for patients on the edge of cirrhosis, with stage 3—or even 4—on the METAVIR fibrosis scale. In Canada, which covers all of its residents' necessary health care, stage 2 had become the norm. Unlike the situation in the U.S., which has a mix of health care payers, in Canada the government usually pays the transplant cost, which varies from province to province. In the U.S. the average cost of a liver transplant, including before and after care, topped $577,000 several years earlier,[1] according to the United Network for Organ Sharing (UNOS), a nonprofit organization that coordinates all types of organ transplants.

It was logical for Canada to avoid transplant expenses by paying even $100,000 for the newest drugs. But at stage F2 on the METAVIR scale in the U.S. or stage F1 in Canada, waiting around with the disease in your system would be unnerving for anyone. Peter Erlinder, director of the International Humanitarian Law Institute in St. Paul, Minnesota, criticized the market-oriented philosophy that had been skewing the standard of care for hepatitis C patients. He compared the availability of Harvoni and Viekira Pak with the Salk and Sabin vaccines. Both the hep C and the polio treatments were cures for a life-threatening disease. Erlinder said the polio vaccines and other breakthroughs such as insulin and penicillin were considered part of America's "social wealth." The government regulated the market to keep prices low. Not so with the $90,000 U.S. price of Harvoni or the $83,000 for Viekira Pak. Many competing hep C drugs have been tested and approved, lowering the price somewhat, for some treatments. Yet the prices have remained stratospheric to the average patient.

In early 2015, when the first non-interferon treatments were being widely prescribed, insurance companies in the United States scrambled to strategize how they would deal with the costly drugs. "The players are flipping out," said Dr. Camilla S. Graham, in an April 2015 webinar for health professionals. Graham is the co-director of the Viral Hepatitis Center at Harvard's Beth Israel Deaconess Medical

Center. Along with insurance companies having to make purchase and coverage decisions for the drugs, Medicaid and Medicare had to grapple with their own sets of rules. Unlike governments in all other countries, the U.S. government was prohibited under law from negotiating prices with pharmaceutical companies. However, most drug companies allow discounts for large public providers. The Veterans Administration usually gets a 40 percent discount on pharmaceuticals, Graham explained in the webinar. Federal prisons get a discount, while state prisons are on their own. Medicaid usually receives a 23 percent rebate off the "best price," according to Graham, but the plan, which helps poor people obtain medical care, varies a lot between states. The system in the U.S. is "phenomenally confusing and complicated," Graham said.

Emalie Huriaux, director of federal and state affairs for Project Inform, a hep C education and advocacy group, used California as an example. The state is about average in its coverage of hepatitis C drugs, she said when I spoke with her in 2015. Its Medicaid program, Medi-Cal, covers antiviral drugs only for people with hep C who are at stage 3 or 4 of liver scarring and have no evidence of substance use.

Some 75 percent of people on Medi-Cal are on Medi-Cal Managed Care, which means that private insurance companies manage their Medi-Cal plan. That causes a disparity in treatment for people with the same disease and the same income. For example, there was an approved Medi-Cal-managed health plan in San Diego County—population over 3 million—that restricted the prescriber to one single hepatologist.

"San Diego County is a huge county," Emalie said. "This has created a huge backlog of hep C patients who are unable to see this provider."

Project Inform had been in touch with an infectious disease specialist in San Diego who had treated hepatitis C for ten years. He is highly skilled at treating people who are coinfected with hep C and HIV, Emalie said, and he gets ten to fifteen referrals of new patients with hepatitis C every week. He has been trying to prescribe the new drugs to his patients. Not one of his patients who scores F3 or F4 on the METAVIR fibrosis scale and qualifies under the Medi-Cal policies has been able to access treatment, Emalie said.

Pauli Gray, a San Francisco Hepatitis C Task Force member whose hep was cured through an AbbVie trial, said a lot of people are falling through the cracks. Gray's day job is with the AIDS Foundation. His clients don't all qualify for treatment for their hepatitis under Medicaid, and they are dealing with HIV, AIDS, and lifestyle problems. "A lot of our clients who have hep C, they don't even care. They have more pressing issues, like a place to sleep," he told me. If the drugs were readily available, his clients would probably get treated, but "the point is," he said, "the drugs are incredibly expensive."

For the more than six hundred private health insurance companies in the United States, costs of the drugs can vary a lot. Some large pharmacies assign a pharmacy benefits manager to negotiate drug prices with the pharmaceutical companies on behalf of the plans. Some insurance companies do their own negotiations. And most insurance companies contain many different plans, which may or may not offer payment for the same drugs to different member groups. In the past, when interferon was the main drug prescribed to hepatitis C patients, insurance companies were less concerned about the cost, presumably because many patients were unwilling to begin or complete a whole course of the dreadful treatment.

The prices the insurance companies negotiate are kept confidential. Erlinder noted that drug wholesalers, the Department of Veterans Affairs, UnitedHealth Group, and other health care providers received discounts of up to 50 percent for Harvoni and Viekira Pak.

But a 50 percent discount on a $90,000 drug still leaves a $45,000 cost. In 2016, almost all private insurance plans in the United States and Canada, as well as U.S. Medicare, Medicaid, and Canadian provincial plans, were rationing hepatitis C treatment to those who had the most advanced liver damage. State-funded care was typically denied until a person was at stage 3—or even cirrhotic at stage 4—on the METAVIR scale. In 2015 Medicaid refused to pay for half of all requests for direct-acting antiviral treatment for hepatitis C, stated Dr. Vincent Lo Re III from the Perelman School of Medicine in a report to the American Association for the Study of Liver Diseases. Canada fared better, with most provinces funding treatment at stage 2.

Today, despite miracle drugs that have become the standard hep C treatment, the high cost is postponing an ultimate, worldwide cure. Yet the pool of people who have been treated with the new drugs has been growing enormously. Thankfully, everyone I spoke with who was infected with hepatitis C when I began writing this book had been cured with direct-acting antivirals by the time the book was completed in early 2017.

Considering the high cure rates and few side effects of the new drugs, Dr. Gary Garber said he can envision hep C vanishing from the world of specialty medicine. "Maybe in three to five years it will be a family doctor kind of treatment," he said in a phone call from Ontario, where he heads infection control for Public Health. "Now with the new medication there's going to be an explosion of people

who would have otherwise not been treated being treated."
The explosion had already started, but some people had
been left out.

Dr. Curtis Cooper summed up the feelings of hepatologists at the 4th Canadian Symposium on Hepatitis C in
Banff, Alberta, in 2015. Cooper, director of the Hepatitis
Program at Ottawa Hospital and associate professor of
infectious diseases at the University of Ottawa, stood in
front of close to three hundred hepatology experts from
throughout the world. Fair-haired and lanky, he appeared
boyish and relaxed. Through a series of slides, he demon-
strated that the rate of hep C infection could slow and new
infections would be gone by 2025 if all patients received
the newest therapies. It would require a commitment by
countries throughout the world to increase their spending on public health, he said. He admitted that would be a
difficult task, calling for research into efficient health care
budgeting. If the costs were to go down significantly, "we'd
treat everybody then. But we also need to be realistic and
reasonable about what we can offer."

I didn't see that as reasonable for many, many people
who were a lot less lucky than me. The demon had blindsided me. The miracle cure had saved me, but more than
100 million people still carried the disease.

I HELD THE clear-packaged gray plastic device and turned
it upside down to examine it. Its handle was the size of a
tongue depressor. Projecting from the handle was a small
plastic spatula with a white, thumbnail-sized tip. Dr. Brian
Conway took another pack from his desk and opened it. He
placed the tip of the device under his tongue and moved it
from one side of his gums to the other. He repeated the action
and plunged the swab into a vial of clear buffer solution.

He placed the antibody tester at the side of his desk as we talked in his office at the Vancouver Infectious Diseases Centre. The office walls were orange. The room held a bookcase, books, and organized clutter, including Brian's medical degree from McGill University, a picture of his graduating class, a friendly greeting card, and a graceful, blooming orchid on top of the bookcase.

Dr. Conway runs the ENTENTE Program out of the clinic. ENTENTE—which stands for "engage, test, engage, treat, and engage"—is funded by the Canadian Institutes of Health Research, along with pharmaceutical companies doing drug trials. Under ENTENTE, medical personnel from the infectious disease clinic travel to outreach events in Vancouver's shabbiest neighborhoods. There Dr. Conway meets IV drug users who are infected with HCV. Typically, on a Friday afternoon, he will travel with a team of five assistants to a community center or gathering point in the Downtown Eastside, places where poor and homeless people watch movies, obtain food, or access services. Dr. Conway offers them the hepatitis C antibody test.

"I'm there with my team and I say, 'People like you often have hepatitis C and they don't know it. So what I'm going to offer you is the opportunity to find out if you have hepatitis C. I'm not going to draw your blood. I'm not going to do anything but put a swab in your mouth,'" he explained as we waited for his own test to complete.

While people attending the outreach program wait, he asks them what kind of services they need. His team will help them fill out subsidized housing or nutritional supplement program forms, or it will direct them toward other outreach programs. He says he has always been motivated to help people in poor communities because life has been unfair to marginalized people. "Somebody has to do something, and it might as well be me," he said.

Fifteen minutes had elapsed. He checked the readout, a white strip embedded under clear plastic on the handle of the OraQuick HCV Rapid Antibody Test. The "C" line was red, indicating the test was complete. The "T" line was empty, indicating that Dr. Conway has never been infected with hepatitis C. A red "T" line would mean hep C antibodies had been found and the patient should undergo an antigen test. Some 20 percent of patients (and 40 percent of Indigenous women)[2] with a "T" line would have developed the antibodies during the acute stage of hepatitis C and fought off the virus then and there, Dr. Conway said. Those whose antigen tests show a viral load would have the chronic virus and could be treated.

At the Infectious Diseases Centre, Dr. Conway doesn't wait for the antigen test. When patients come to see him there and learn they have antibodies to hepatitis C, they can immediately get a FibroScan at the clinic. If it shows significant fibrosis, Dr. Conway will work to quickly get them treatment. If the fibrosis level is low, he counsels them or helps them enroll in programs that might pay for their drugs before stage 2—and provincial funding—kicks in.

"It's wonderful that you do that," I said to Dr. Conway. "But what about people like me, who aren't part of the marginalized population, who come to your clinic?"

"That's a different group," he said. He said poor and addicted patients, like those he generally sees, constitute only half of those who have been diagnosed with hepatitis C in Canada. The rest are people like me, mostly baby boomers, whose hepatitis started in their youth, in the days of experimentation when fun often equaled foolishness.

Some people don't remember that they were exposed to any risk factors, Dr. Conway said, and they're unlikely to show up in one of his mobile clinics. The solution would be to test all baby boomers, he said.

In the United States, the Centers for Disease Control has recognized that, and recommends that all people born between 1945 and 1965 be tested for HCV at least once. Health Canada has called only for risk-based screening. The Canadian Liver Foundation wants those born from 1945 through 1975 to be tested and has a risk-assessment tool on its website. If people see a problem, they should get tested. However, it seems unlikely that most people with early-stage liver disease who feel no symptoms will ever visit the site.

Daryl Luster, the president of the Pacific Hepatitis C Network, sees the U.S. vision of testing as an ideal. "Seventy-five to 80 percent of the people now living with hep C are baby boomers. They're just hanging around getting sicker and sicker," he said. He has been pushing for testing of all baby boomers since 2012, but when I met with him at a Starbucks in 2014, he had become uncertain about his stance. The data supported it, he said. "I believe in data. I believe in science, but what I am hearing is 'Don't promote testing because we can't treat them [people with hep C].' Is it ethical to promote testing if we're not going to treat them?"

I had been tested by chance, and then, like a typical optimistic baby boomer, I had believed the antibodies in my blood proved that hepatitis had come and gone. More than a month had elapsed before I learned that twenty thousand hepatitis C RNA particles infected every milliliter of my blood. I lagged in arranging doctor's appointments, and my trip to Mexico postponed my diagnosis. In the long run, for me, that didn't matter too much. But for thousands of others, a small delay can mean a difference between life and death. Hepatitis C continues to attack the liver until the virus is gone. At a certain point the damage may become irreversible. Like hockey player Bill Demish, many thousands of people, while they waited for treatment, have had their liver move from the early stages of fibrosis to advanced, serious liver scarring. A time lag before diagnosis can be deadly too. In some cases, especially in underequipped parts of the world, delays are often a matter of money. Some impoverished people can't even get started on the road to a cure.

Scientist and medical doctor Jordan Feld teaches at the University of Toronto medical school and lectures around the world about advances in hepatology. He works with a team of five laboratory researchers and twenty clinicians at the Sandra Rotman Centre, which tackles pernicious global diseases, including hepatitis C. In some developing countries, direct-acting antivirals that can cure hepatitis C are inexpensive, whereas tests that uncover the infection are not, Feld said. As a result, people may not get treated, simply because they haven't been tested. "In many impoverished countries, testing is key to getting any treatment at all," he said. "Fewer than 10% and possibly fewer than 5% of the over 100 million people with Hep C have been diagnosed worldwide. It's pretty staggering," Feld exclaimed in an email in October 2016.

When all is said and done, the best and certainly the permanent cure for hepatitis C worldwide would be to stop its spread everywhere in the world. That means at the least that every person with even the slightest risk should be tested. It also means that anyone who tests positive should be immediately treated, and that no one who has the disease should pass it on to anyone else. Daryl Luster suggests starting with "a really aggressive, robust plan" for harm reduction among the 15 percent of people with hepatitis C who currently use IV drugs. Those marginalized patients are among the group Dr. Conway treats. He is sometimes able to get payment approval for the high-cost direct-acting antivirals for addicts even when they have minimal fibrosis—because there is so great a risk they will pass hepatitis C to someone else.

At the same time, millions of baby boomers are decades past the days of their perhaps isolated incidents of IV drug use, risky sex, tattoo embellishment, unscreened blood transfusions, or other means of hep C transmission. They are now realtors or retired machinists or CEOs. They have hep C but don't know it. They are unlikely to pass it on to someone else, and they may also be unlikely to be treated. Maybe a CEO can pay for a $1,000-per-pill drug, but the auto mechanic with a wife, two kids, and a steep mortgage cannot. Just a few years ago, many people opted to wait for treatment because the treatment was often worse than the disease. But today, given the ease of taking Harvoni, Viekira Pak, Zepatier, and other non-interferon antivirals and the speed with which they work, once a person knows the demon has entered their blood, they want to immediately annihilate it.

Dr. Curtis Cooper and I talked on the phone about the situation. "The new treatments represent therapy that almost everybody can take safely and tolerate well, which really represents a huge leap forward. But it comes with a big price tag," he said. "Ideally, I would treat everybody as soon as they came through my door, but we need to put our priorities somewhere, and that needs to be people with more advanced liver disease. But it's hard for a person to live with a chronic disease. They feel stigmatized. Some people feel like they're a lesser human or they're dirty. It's tough to live with that, especially with the knowledge that there's treatment that can eliminate reinfection."

But even if the price of the drugs were to drop a thousandfold, that goal will remain a fantasy if people fail to get tested.

AT THE END of my treatment, I was confident that my hep C had vanished, but I was equally sure my liver had been damaged. The virus had driven it perilously close to if not into cirrhosis. According to the nurses I had overheard talking about my FibroScan results, my liver had been either at the top of stage 3 fibrosis or at the bottom of stage 4, which is cirrhosis. If my liver were to remain badly scarred, I would worry for the rest of my life. I would abstain from drinking even a drop of alcohol, from downing Tylenol for a headache, and from eating any kind of fatty food, for fear of doing more harm. I hoped my liver would at least become healthy enough so that someday I could join in a friend's birthday celebration or a New Year's toast with a glass of champagne.

But the champagne would have to wait. On New Year's 2015 I still didn't know the state of my liver. After hep C is cured, some—though not all—livers regress to an earlier stage. Maria said many of her patients surprised her when their post-treatment livers regressed to a lower stage on the METAVIR scale. It could happen to anyone, she said, and she mentioned an elderly woman patient of hers whose liver had regressed to stage 1 from cirrhosis. Dr. Ramji, however, took the glass-half-empty approach. Liver regression doesn't happen to everyone, he warned me. It is unpredictable. So while I was relieved to have vanquished the demon,

I remained on edge about my health. Statistics didn't help. A 2002 study in the journal *Gastroenterology* looked at three thousand patients who had endured interferon treatment for hepatitis C. Biopsies performed twenty months after the beginning of their treatment showed they averaged only a 20 percent chance of regression of at least one stage. There was no change in 65 percent of the test subjects and an increase in fibrosis in 15 percent.

Recent studies of patients treated with direct-acting antivirals are more promising. In 2014 researchers from the Akron General Medical Center looked at six studies and found that given time, even patients with cirrhosis are likely to experience some regression.

If cirrhosis progresses into end-stage liver disease, only a liver transplant can save you. Yet the liver can function well even when only part of it is intact, and transplant livers can come from living donors. About half of the donor's liver is removed during surgery. Within eight to twelve weeks both the donor's and the recipient's livers are expected to almost completely regenerate to full size and function.

I thought of this one day when I was relaxing on my deck with my two daughters. They are different in personality and appearance from each other, but both are successful, poised, creative, congenial, philosophical women. As I talked with them, the sun shone brightly, sending glints onto the ocean below. We shaded ourselves under a patio umbrella and sipped tea. I explained I was probably cured but had no idea about the state of my liver.

"I'll give you a piece of my liver," said Della. "I will too," Jessica said.

# EPILOGUE

B Y LATE 2016, more than two years after my cure, the outlook on hepatitis C had changed. At the beginning of the year around a dozen oral direct-acting antivirals and many combination treatments had either recently been approved or were in trials for hepatitis C. Conferences on the disease increasingly lumped it with hepatitis B, calling the health problem "viral hepatitis." Hep C could be cured with near absolute certainty—for those who knew they had it—yet a cure for the B virus had eluded scientists.

Since the time of my treatment, issues over the cost and coverage of hep C drugs have continued and have prompted lawsuits. Among these was a class action suit filed against Gilead Sciences on behalf of the Southeastern Pennsylvania Transportation Authority. The suit claimed that Sovaldi's excessive price violated the Sherman Antitrust Act and the Affordable Care Act. Two prisoners filed a lawsuit against Minnesota's Department of Corrections for refusing to fund their hep C treatment. There were also a number of lawsuits by individuals against insurance companies that had denied them coverage for direct-acting antivirals.

Entire countries were embroiled in the cost problem. Sweden's universal pharmacare system, in which patients pay only $350 a year for their drugs, was contemplating restrictions on coverage. It had seen a 6 percent uptick in yearly drug costs in 2014–15, mostly attributed to the two top hep C drugs. In addition to China's rejection of the Sovaldi patent, India, Argentina, Brazil, China, Russia, and Ukraine challenged hepatitis C drug patents. The impetus for the challenge was that an unpatented drug could be produced generically and cheaply. Even a U.S. presidential candidate got into the action: in 2016 Democratic presidential hopeful Bernie Sanders called for the Veterans Administration to use emergency powers to bypass patent rules on Gilead and AbbVie hepatitis C drugs.

The U.S. Senate report on the pricing of Sovaldi was released in December 2015. After looking at twenty thousand pages of Gilead company documents and information from Medicaid programs throughout the country, the Senate determined that in twenty-one months, U.S. sales of Sovaldi and Harvoni had totaled $20.6 billion. In a news conference announcing the report, committee member Senator Ron Wyden (D-Oregon) said, "Gilead pursued a calculated scheme for pricing and marketing its Hepatitis C drug based on one primary goal, maximizing revenue, regardless of the human consequences."[1]

In spring 2016, Australia made treatment with direct-acting antivirals available for anyone with hepatitis C, regardless of the degree of liver scarring. The government health plan pays for the meds. Anyone who holds a Medicare card (every Australian citizen gets one) can get a prescription through their family doctor, after the doctor consults with a hepatologist. The Pharmaceuticals Benefit Scheme pays for the drugs, and the patient pays a $6 to $38 dispensing fee.

EVERYONE I SPOKE with during the writing of this book is still alive, though some are faring better than others. The great news is that every one of them who sought treatment for hepatitis C eventually got it.

Andrew Loog Oldham, former manager of the Rolling Stones, who lives part-time in Vancouver, also keeps a home in Colombia, where his wife's family and his adopted street dogs live. While direct-acting antivirals for hepatitis C were undergoing clinical trials, his acupuncturist in Colombia said, "You've been lucky all your life, Andrew. There's a drug coming along that will save the day for you."

Around the time we met for tea in Vancouver, Andrew started treatment with Harvoni. He began writing a book about his illness and talking to community groups about the need to be tested for HCV. In January 2016, the *Globe and Mail* reported that Andrew was free of the hepatitis C virus.

Jim Banta's fall from the scaffolding had led to interferon treatment, which came too late to save his liver. A transplant saved his life. Throughout his journey, his wife and two sons were incredible, he said: "They've been through wars with me. I'm a pretty lucky guy." Jim became an ambassador for the California Transplant Donor Network (now Donor Network West). He's on the San Francisco Hep C Task Force and facilitates hepatitis C support groups.

After a seven-year wait, artist Anahid Aslanyan began twelve weeks of Harvoni, which she finished in February 2015. Her virus cleared in the second week and has stayed clear ever since. In fall 2015 her fibrosis remained at stage 3 on the METAVIR scale. She was optimistic that in a couple of years her liver would regress. Anahid exhibits her paintings frequently at gallery shows.

Ben Handley's partner, Dennis Ronson, underwent Harvoni treatment in 2015. He was free of hepatitis C by that summer. The couple hoped a cure for HIV will be discovered.

John Lavette started treatment with Harvoni on Valentine's Day 2015. By the end of summer he was clear of hep. As always, he makes people laugh with tales of sex and adventure in his hippie days.

Dr. Ramji sent musician Adam Bailey for a FibroScan, which revealed that his liver was at stage 3. That was enough to initiate insurance coverage. Harvoni treatment caused fatigue, so Adam took time off work. By October 2015 he was back installing home automation devices and clear of hepatitis C.

The doctor who had managed computer techie Shirley Barger's failed clinical trial continued doing studies at the California Pacific Medical Center. He and his colleagues felt bad about her misery with the squirming pencil-like DUROS device, Shirley said. "I think it actually served me well and made me memorable to the doctors, so they would consider me when something good came along."

She was invited into another trial, which studied a one-pill combination of GS-5885, a NS5A protein inhibitor, and sofosbuvir. Later, the numbered drug was named ledipasvir, and eventually the combination was called Harvoni. It cured her. She was appointed to the San Francisco Hepatitis C Task Force and is on the advisory board of the *HCV Advocate*. She reported in February 2016 that twelve people in the support group she leads had been cured by direct-acting antivirals.

Bill Demish is now in his eighties and still loves hockey.

Prestige Health Choice denied my niece Sandy's appeal for funding of Harvoni. By the end of 2015, her insurance company had refused four separate applications for treatment, my sister Mary reported. Mary asked Gilead's Support Path program to subsidize Sandy's antivirals, but the program said it would help only with an insurance co-payment. Because the insurer denied coverage, there was no support.

By 2016 insurers in the United States had begun to reduce their fibrosis-level restrictions. That year costs fell significantly with the FDA's approval of Merck's drug Zepatier ($54,600 for a twelve-week treatment). As the summer of 2016 wound down, Mary planned to apply on Sandy's behalf for insurance coverage for the new drug, but before she did, she got a call from Sandy's gastroenterologist's office. An intake person asked Mary to bring Sandy to the office so she could be shown how to use Harvoni. Mary worried that the drug was being prescribed because Sandy's fibrosis might have climbed over stage 3 and become very serious.

That wasn't the case. In a treatment room on September 2, 2016, nurse practitioner Angel Adams assured Mary that Sandy was still at stage 2. She gave Mary a thirty-day supply of Harvoni to begin Sandy's treatment. When Mary got home that day she wrote about the encounter with Angel to me in an email:

> I expressed my astonishment again and asked her how this had come about. She told me, "We have many, many patients just like Sandy who have been denied medication." It seems the CDC told the insurance companies when the drug first came out, "You're going to be flooded

with demands for this drug so please make sure you treat the sickest ones first." The insurance companies (to their own advantage) interpreted this to mean "Treat only the sickest ones." Apparently, many people who were denied treatment appealed to the CDC. They in turn pressured the insurance companies to treat everyone who was sick.

So it seemed to me that the USA was on its way to treating everyone who has hepatitis C. As for Sandy, by January 2017 she was hep free—and her liver had regressed to normal.

AT THE BEGINNING of treatment, my liver thumped at 12.7, which was on the border of cirrhosis. Twelve weeks after my last dose of antivirals, my fibrosis thumped at 4.9. A full year after treatment, my FibroScan score had dipped to 3.9, which is METAVIR stage 0 to 1. On May 3, 2016, a reading of 3.2 appeared on the FibroScan screen. "Your liver's healthy," Dr. Ramji said. "You won't need to see me again, or at least not for a very long time."

I talked with my sister Irene again, but neither of us apologized.

I never sent the letter to Dr. Halliman.

THE MONTH AFTER I split up with Peter, the United States declared amnesty for war resisters. I pleaded with him to go home. After he repeatedly burst into my friend Sonya's home, where I was living, and after I was forced to move out because of his rages, Peter returned to New York. I never saw him after that.

I recently learned what happened to him. As I write this, I'm still in shock. While I was fact-checking this book, I thought I should check one last thing. I had learned from a genealogist that Peter had died in 2011—in Arizona, of all places. I wanted to know what had happened. I was no longer Peter's immediate relative, so I asked Jessica, his biological daughter, to send for his death certificate. It arrived less than a week before I submitted the manuscript of this book to the publisher.

I opened the envelope in my kitchen and pulled out a folded sheet of paper. It was full of boxes, full of fine print. There was scrollwork at the top and an Arizona state seal at the bottom. I read some short lines of text and gasped. I grabbed the edge of the counter for balance. The document stated:

Immediate cause of death: hepatic failure
Due to or as a consequence of: hepatic cirrhosis
Other significant conditions contributing to death: hepatitis C

The mystery remains.

# ACKNOWLEDGMENTS

I WANT TO THANK, first and foremost, my immediate family. My husband, Al, was a solid, constant support throughout my treatment for hepatitis. When I was first diagnosed and was frightened about my infection, he encouraged me to ease my mind through writing. Most importantly, when I was ready to cry, he made me laugh, which influenced the tone of this book. It started as a serious, academic look at a serious disease, but Al's ability to analyze the social side of any issue prompted me to shape it as much as possible into a conversation with the reader. When the book was in the editing stage, Al read through it and gave me solid, incredibly helpful advice.

I have been blessed with having wonderful, kindhearted children who grew to be wonderful, kindhearted, successful adults. Their comfort and friendship gave me strength throughout my struggle with hepatitis C. In this book you met my oldest daughter as a preschooler. I thank Della immensely for the memories I have of her that became part of my story. She has inspired me since the day she was born, two days before I turned eighteen. You met my younger daughter, Jessica Raya, right after she was born. While I was writing this book, she was working on her second novel, *Prayers for Pyros* (McClelland & Stewart, 2017). She took time off from that huge task and read through the more personal parts of my narrative. Her feedback helped and encouraged me greatly. Both of my daughters were always in my heart as I wrote.

My thanks go to the many doctors and researchers who talked with me about hepatitis issues. Doctors Jordan Feld, Curtis Cooper, Brian Conway, and Gary Garber were especially helpful with current developments in hepatitis C research. So was the team of health professionals who guided me through my personal journey with hep: Dr. Iris Radev, Dr. Alnoor Ramji, and clinical research manager Maria Ancheta-Schmidt. Thanks also to Misha Cohen, for her useful advice on Chinese medicine. Not only did all of these people provide needed information for this book, but they also explained many concepts about the disease in simple terms. A writer loves to hear those kinds of explanations. Dr. Feld gets an extra special five-star thank-you for expertly checking facts in this book about the hep C virus and the liver. He's a busy clinician-scientist who saves a lot of lives through his work, and he graciously took the time to help me. He reviewed many but not all of the facts. If there are any mistakes, they are mine, not his.

Maria Ancheta-Schmidt and Dr. Iris Radev also get my thanks for being angels. That's my designation for ten special women who inspired me to write even when I was most distressed about my disease. Among these angels were friends and neighbors who were my most frequent confidants. They each listened with an open heart when I talked about my infection, and they asked questions that helped me determine what readers would want to know. My thanks go to Shannon, Marilyn, Sophie, Shelley, Marla, Susan, and Jen. Rounding off the angel list is Allison Waithe, who filled me in on patient support programs and comforted me when I was most anxious about treatment. All of these angel women helped immeasurably (although they didn't know it) to smooth out the tone of this book and to give me confidence in writing it.

A great pile of thanks goes to my editor, Nancy Flight, a longtime friend who cheered me while I was in the throes of my disease. She steered me toward shaping this book for readers like you, and she took on all of the book's complexity as an editor. She made the book much better than I could ever have managed by myself.

My publisher, Rob Sanders, was also instrumental in making this book what it is. He trusted me to take on this project and to finish it quickly. Moreover, he gets my thanks for suggesting that I dig into my past to describe what happened when I was infected with hepatitis C. That small suggestion sent me into periods of deep thought about my life as a child, as a teenager, and as a young adult, and it helped me discover long-buried incidents that shed light on how I may have acquired the virus.

Huge thanks go to my agent, Robert Lecker, for being knowledgeable and clear in dealing with all the intricacies involved in making a book proposal work. Robert also gets a big star for probably being the quickest person in Canada in responding to email. Robert, you are amazing!

As I was writing this book, I ran into a friend I hadn't seen in more than a decade. Judith Comfort had been an author and a teacher-librarian. She moved to the Sunshine Coast and took up genealogy, which proved invaluable in my writing of this book—and led to its surprising ending, which shocked me more than I can express. Judith wowed me with the speed and depth of her research. My deepest gratitude goes to her for her help.

I also reconnected with two of my favorite teaching colleagues, Abbe Nielsen and Cheryl McKeeman. They helped me dredge up memories of a kayak trip we took many years ago. Many, many thanks to them for sharing their excellent recollection of a day when I was too weary to save the details in my mind.

Thanks go to some wonderful people from San Francisco who shared information about hepatitis C. I'd like to thank Emalie Huriaux, director of federal and state affairs for Project Inform, and Shirley Barger of the San Francisco Hepatitis C Task Force. They both helped me connect with many other people involved in hepatitis C advocacy. Emalie provided much-needed information on the ability of hep C patients to access treatment. Shirley told me the harrowing story of her own years of treatment. Pauli Gray, another San Francisco Hepatitis C Task Force member, supplied valuable information as well. Emalie, Shirley, and Pauli get my deepest thanks.

I also send my thanks to the many people who shared the stories of their journeys with hepatitis C. Jim Banta, also a San Francisco Task Force member, Ben Handley, John Lavette, Adam Bailey, Nita Rippin, and Bill Demish get my heartfelt appreciation. They were all wonderfully sincere and gracious. A couple of people spent a huge amount of time telling their stories to me. John Lavette was charming, funny, and talkative. He has so many anecdotes to tell that I could write a movie about his life. That's fitting because when John's not filling San Francisco with flowers, he's an actor. Anahid Aslanyan also contributed an enormous amount of time sharing her story and helping me with information for this book. When I needed a break, I often went to her website (http://anahida-creations.weebly.com/) to look at her art. It inspired me as I wrote. Anahid, I love your artwork.

A special thank-you goes to Andrew Loog Oldham, former manager of the Rolling Stones, who was both gracious and candid in telling me the story of his hepatitis C infection. When I met with him, he was six or seven chapters into shaping his own book about his experience with hepatitis C. Not all authors writing their own book about a topic would share their experiences with another author working on a similar idea. I can't wait to read your book, Andrew.

While writing this book I was in frequent contact with my sister Mary Rudolf-Helvaty. Unending thanks go to Mary and my niece Sandy for coming forward with their story and giving me immense help in many, many ways. They live three thousand miles away from me, but their help in my work on this book made me feel like they were right next door.

As well, I'd like to thank the many hepatitis C support and advocacy groups that helped me gather and confirm information for this book. A big heap of appreciation goes to Daryl Luster, the president of the Pacific Hepatitis C Network. Daryl does a superb job of shining light on the need for testing and treatment. He provided valuable insights into the state of hepatitis C care, and he inspired me with his optimism.

Many people opened up to me with their stories but for understandable reasons asked that their names be withheld. They had jobs to lose or other issues that kept me from revealing their identities. The stories they shared with me are every bit as appreciated as every other contributor's to this book.

Also my thanks go to the dozens of other people who contacted me with their knowledge and stories. This book was written on a tight deadline, and I was not able to get back to everyone. But I was amazed and thankful for the overwhelming response to my request for interviews.

In writing this book I read through scores of research studies on hepatitis C topics. Most of them had many authors, and each study represents weeks or months or years of their work. My thanks go to every single one of those dedicated people. A number of the studies are cited in the Selected Notes and References section of this book. The full list of references is available on my website at www.rains.ca. I've tried to include every researcher's name. If I missed anyone, they get a double thank-you.

The subject matter of this book was complex. I sought help from experts and tried to simplify information for easy reading. Occasionally, two or more studies I cited showed differing results, but that's not unreasonable, given variations in test subjects and conditions. If I mis-stated anything, readers should keep in mind that I'm not a doctor. For exact explanations about hepatitis C and the science around it, they should talk with medical personnel who specialize in the disease. Also, some topics changed as I wrote about them, particularly issues surrounding drug costs. I hope that in time some of what I've written becomes history and costs come down and testing goes up, so that everyone with hepatitis C can be treated.

# MY GOOD FOR THE LIVER LIST

YOU CAN LIVE with an artificial heart, but you can't live without your liver. It's the largest internal organ and performs the body's most complex work. It deserves to be pampered with these foods. They are ordered according to a list I hung from my refrigerator until months after I was cured of hepatitis C. Water is at the top because of its importance, but the rest are in random order.

**Water**
Drink lots. Our bodies contain up to 60 percent water. With the help of the liver, water cleanses the body of waste and toxins. If you find water boring, squeeze a lemon into a glass of it and read on.

**Citrus Fruit**
Lemons, oranges, and grapefruit contain high amounts of vitamin C, which helps the body break down toxins.

Citrus fruit also contains flavonoids. These water-soluble, brightly colored nutrients can reduce inflammation associated with hepatitis C. The lemon flavonoid hesperidin has been shown to protect the liver against toxicity. Oranges are high in vitamin A, an antioxidant that guards against free radicals, which can hasten liver cancer for those with cirrhosis. Grapefruit contains the flavonoid naringenin, which may inhibit hep C's secretion from cells, but check to see if the fruit is compatible with any medications you are taking. Avoid sugary fruit drinks, since concentrated sugar may stress the digestive process and the liver.

### Coffee
My mother, who lived to be ninety-nine years old, drank at least eight cups of coffee a day (no kidding) for at least fifty years. Need I say more? But I will. Study after study has shown that coffee can lessen liver damage from hepatitis C. An analysis of all studies on the topic between 1986 and 2012 indexed on MEDLINE and PubMed (two of the most comprehensive websites for the medical professions) revealed that drinking three or more cups a day beneficially affects enzyme levels and decreases the progression of cirrhosis. Most people know that too much coffee can cause sleeplessness and indigestion. Try three cups a day, all before noon.

### Avocados
This fruit (some people call it a vegetable) helps the body produce glutathione, which the liver uses for detoxification. Researchers in Japan found that five compounds in avocados reduced liver damage in rats. To give your liver an extra boost of good stuff, eat a plain avocado drenched in lemon juice.

### Apples

Pectin, a soluble fiber found in the cell walls of plants, is particularly high in apples and helps remove toxins from the blood. The apple flavonoid phlorizin can aid the liver by stimulating bile production. An apple a day may keep liver damage at bay.

### Leafy Green Vegetables

Spinach, kale, collard greens, dark green lettuce, and even young dandelion leaves can remove toxins from the bloodstream. Green leafy vegetables are known to neutralize nasty chemicals, including pesticides. The less bad stuff that goes into the liver, the less work the liver will have to do, and the more resources it will maintain to fight hepatitis.

### Sulfur-Containing Bulbs

Garlic, onions, shallots, and leeks all contain pungent sulfur compounds. The sulfur compound in garlic, allicin, helps rid the body of mercury, estrogen, and some food additives. Onions, shallots, and leeks help the liver produce glutathione, which aids the liver's cleansing activities.

### Broccoli, Brussels Sprouts, Cabbage, and Cauliflower

Cruciferous vegetables, including these four, are good sources of glucosinolate, a sulfur-containing compound that becomes pungent when chewed. More than three studies show that glucosinolate reduces cholesterol levels and prevents disease. Cabbage helps activate two liver-detoxifying enzymes. Unfortunately, a sniff of boiled cabbage reminds me of a dank piece of cloth. To avoid the wet-cloth smell, try eating cabbage kimchi, coleslaw, cabbage soup, and sauerkraut.

## Turmeric

You see this yellow spice in virtually every book and website that gives diet advice to people stricken with hepatitis C. Turmeric contains enzymes that flush carcinogens from the liver.

## Walnuts

Walnuts contain the amino acid arginine, which detoxifies ammonia. They are also a good source of glutathione and omega-3 fatty acids. While being treated for hepatitis C, I kept a jar of walnuts in my pantry and often grabbed a few for a snack.

## Eggs

During my ordeal with hepatitis C, I began each day with an egg. It was comfort food to me, but eggs also contain choline, which protects the liver from toxins and heavy metals. The Mayo Clinic says an egg a day does little to increase the risk of heart disease. Just avoid bacon or sausages on the side.

# SELECTED NOTES
# AND REFERENCES

IN RESEARCHING THIS book, I consulted dozens of books, hundreds of studies, and many experts. The original manuscript contained twenty-seven pages of footnotes. After consulting with my publisher, I moved most of them to my website. That allows more detail and lets me update web addresses if they change. Below are some notes readers may want to view initially, including sources for quotes. For the full set of notes and references—as well as information on hepatitis C—please see www.rains.ca/demon.

**Introduction**

1. Governments, health organizations, and at least one multinational drug manufacturer announced plans to eliminate the virus entirely.

   In 2016 Georgia (a former part of the USSR) announced a hepatitis C elimination policy and Scotland debated elimination in its parliament (both cited in many news reports). The European

Union HCV Summit in Brussels on February 17, 2016, announced
elimination plans; see the webcast at http://www.natap.org/2016/
HCV/021916_05.htm. Also see Catherine Jewell, "Gilead Targets
Elimination of Hepatitis C," *WIPO Magazine,* World Intellectual
Property Organization (February 2015), 2–5.

### Chapter 1

1. The U.S. Army reports that doctors in the '20s and '30s noticed
   "epidemic jaundice."
   The U.S. Army Medical Department, Office of Medical History,
   provides extensive documentation on the history of hepatitis.
   This quote can be found in Joe A. Dean and Andre J. Ognibene,
   "Hepatitis," chapter 18 in *Internal Medicine in Vietnam,* Vol. 2, *General Medicine and Infectious Diseases,* edited by Andre J. Ognibene
   and O'Neill Barrett, Jr. (Washington, DC: Office of the Surgeon
   General and Center of Military History, United States Army,
   1982), http://history.amedd.army.mil/booksdocs/vietnam/
   GenMedvN/ch18.html.

### Chapter 2

1. According to July 2016 figures from the World Health Organization, hepatitis C infects up to 150 million people...
   World Health Organization statistics state that 130 to 150 million
   people are infected with hepatitis C; World Health Organization,
   "Hepatitis C Fact Sheet," July 2016, http://www.who.int/media-
   centre/factsheets/fs164/en/. As more and more people received
   the new antivirals, WHO issued a "Global Report on Access to
   Hepatitis C Treatment" in October 2016 that stated, "Estimates
   of the number of people living with hepatitis C infection vary
   widely," and could be as low as 80 million for the chronic disease.

**Chapter 3**

1. The study concluded that there is a "theoretical risk of infection by sharing these objects."
   G. Lock, M. Dirscherl, F. Obermeier, C.M. Gelbmann, C. Hellerbrand, A. Knöll, J. Schölmerich, and W. Jilg, "Hepatitis C Contamination of Toothbrushes: Myth or Reality?" *Journal of Viral Hepatitis* 13, no. 9 (September 2006): 571–73, doi: 10.1111/j.1365-2893.2006.00735.x.

2. "The mere finding of HCV-RNA on the surface…"
   Lock et al., "Hepatitis C Contamination of Toothbrushes."

3. Egypt's vaccination campaign used contaminated needles and syringes…
   World Health Organization, "Egypt Steps Up Efforts against Hep C," July 2014, http://www.who.int/features/2014/egypt-campaign-hepatitisc/en/.

4. Vietnam is also high on the World Health Organization's hepatitis C crisis list…
   National Institutes of Health, "Jenny Heathcote," *Great Teachers: Treating Chronic Hepatitis B and C,* Clinical Grand Rounds, video, January 13, 2013, http://videocast.nih.gov/Summary.asp?File=15539&bhcp=1.

5. "An investigator probably said, 'Oh isn't that interesting?…'"
   Dr. Gary Garber did not specifically name the clinics that were connected with the infections. We spoke about the hep C outbreak on April 8, 2015, and again during fact-checking.

6. The investigation turned up another three infected patients who had visited the Tri-City Colonoscopy Clinic…
   The specific mention of the Tri-City Colonoscopy Clinic comes from "Hepatitis C Outbreak Identified at Kitchener Colonoscopy Clinic," CBC News, February 3, 2015, http://www.cbc.ca/news/canada/kitchener-waterloo/hepatitis-c-outbreak-identified-at-kitchener-colonoscopy-clinic-1.2943603.

**Chapter 5**

1.  Yet I shudder to contemplate the sketchy treatments some people like Johnny with hep C undergo.

    I've consulted extensive studies on conventional medical treatment for hepatitis C, but some of the self-treatment methods and cures in this chapter are not backed by peer-reviewed studies. I'm referring mainly to Johnny Delirious's self-treatments and am not suggesting that anyone try them. I wrote about Delirious to show the extent some people go to when trying to cure their own hepatitis C.

2.  ... transmission of hepatitis C occurs in only one out of 190,000 sexual encounters.

    Norah A. Terrault, Jennifer L. Dodge, Edward L. Murphy, John E. Tavis, Alexi Kiss, T.R. Levin, Robert G. Gish, Michael P. Busch, Arthur L. Reingold, and Miriam J. Alter, "Sexual Transmission of Hepatitis C Virus among Monogamous Heterosexual Couples: The HCV Partners Study," *Hepatology* 57, no. 3 (March 2013): 881–89, doi: 10.1002/hep.26164.

3.  ... an early direct-acting antiviral for hepatitis C, boceprevir, was associated with priapism.

    Kyle P. Hammond, Craig Nielsen, Sunny A. Linnebur, Jacob A. Langness, Graham Ray, Paul Maroni, and Jennifer J. Kiser, "Priapism Induced by Boceprevir-CYP3A4 Inhibition and Alpha-Adrenergic Blockade: Case Report," *Clinical Infectious Diseases* 58, no. 1 (January 2014): e35–38, doi: 10.1093/cid/cit673.

**Chapter 6**

1.  Between 40 and 75 percent of people who have hepatitis C don't know they have it.

    This wide range was given because of differing figures from U.S. and Canadian sources. The Centers for Disease Control and Prevention in the United States states that up to three out of four people who are infected with hepatitis C don't know it; Centers for Disease Control and Prevention, "Hepatitis C: Testing Baby Boomers Saves Lives," *CDC Vitalsigns,* May 2013, http://www.cdc.gov/vitalsigns/hepatitisc/. The Public Health Agency of Canada says that 40 percent of people with hepatitis C don't know they have it; Public Health Agency of Canada, "Hepatitis C: Get the Facts," March 2, 2015, http://www.phac-aspc.gc.ca/hepc/pubs/getfacts-informezvous/index-eng.php.

2. ... one out of thirty baby boomers is afflicted with the virus.
   Centers for Disease Control and Prevention, "CDC Now Recommends All Baby Boomers Receive One-Time Hepatitis C Test," press release, August 26, 2012.

3. The study suggests that brain fog is a chronic effect of the virus and not a permanent change in the brain.
   Marco Senzolo, Sami Schiff, Cristina Maria D'Aloiso, Chiara Crivellin, Evangelos Cholongitas, Patrizia Burra, and Sara Montagnese, "Neuropsychological Alterations in Hepatitis C Infection: The Role of Inflammation," *World Journal of Gastroenterology* 17, no. 29 (August 7, 2011): 3369–74, doi: 10.3748/wjg.v17.i29.3369.

4. "As of April 2001, based on a Public Health Advisory issued in the U.S ..."
   Page Novartis, "Important Drug Safety Information," at Government of Canada, Healthy Canadians, "Archived—Important Drug Warning—Lamisil—(Terbinafine HCL)—Novartis," May 17, 2001, http://healthycanadians.gc.ca/recall-alert-rappel-avis/hc-sc/2001/14531a-eng.php.

5. Intarcia Therapeutics, which sponsored the trial of Omega DUROS therapy...
   Intarcia Therapeutics, Inc. explained trial results of Omega DUROS therapy in a press release: "Intarcia Therapeutics Announces Final Results from a Phase 2 Study of Injectable Omega Interferon Plus Ribavirin for the Treatment of Hepatitis C Genotype-1," April 12, 2012, http://www.intarcia.com/media/press-releases/2007-apr-12-injectable-omega.html.

## Chapter 7

1. The problems with interferon...

   The statistics come from Peter Loftus, "Patient Dilemma: Treat
   Hepatitis C Now or Hold Out?" *Wall Street Journal,* March 4,
   2013, http://www.wsj.com/articles/SB10001424127887323293
   704578330712442353712. Loftus gave a 40 to 45 percent initial cure rate for interferon, but some sources put this closer to
   50 percent.

## Chapter 8

1. In 2016, insurance companies in the U.S. were getting about a
   45 percent discount...

   Associated Press, "FDA OKs Merck Hepatitis C Drug, Adding to
   Patient Choices," *Modern Healthcare,* January 29, 2016, http://
   www.modernhealthcare.com/article/20160129/NEWS/160129841.

2. ... the drug could be produced for less than $2 a pill.

   Based on an estimate of $68 to $136 for a twelve-week supply of
   sofosbuvir in Andrew Will, Saye Khoo, Joe Fortunak, Bryony
   Simmons, and Nathan Ford, "Minimum Costs for Producing
   Hepatitis C Direct Acting Antivirals, for Use in Large-Scale
   Treatment Access Programs in Developing Countries," *Clinical
   Infectious Diseases* 58, no. 7 (April 2014): 928–36, doi: 10.1093/
   cid/ciu012.

## Chapter 10

1. "Your request does not meet pharmacy coverage guidelines..."
   Prestige Health Choice, letter to Sandy Rudolf, July 9, 2015.

## Chapter 11

1. In the U.S. the average cost of a liver transplant, including before
   and after care, topped $577,000 several years ago...
   It probably costs more today, but there were no current
   amounts available at the time of writing. This is a 2011 figure

($577,100) from UNOS Transplant Living, https://web.archive.
org/web/20150319015437/http://transplantliving.org/
before-the-transplant/financing-a-transplant/the-costs/.

2. ... (and 40 percent of Indigenous women)...
Dr. Conway coauthored a study that found a high rate of hepati-
tis C clearance among Indigenous women: Jason Grebely, Jesse
D. Raffa, Calvin Lai, Mel Krajden, Brian Conway, and Mark
W. Tyndall, "Factors Associated with Spontaneous Clearance
of Hepatitis C Virus among Illicit Drug Users," *Canadian
Journal of Gastroenterology* 21, no. 7 (July 2007): 447–51, doi:
10.1155/2007/796325.

**Epilogue**

1. "Gilead pursued a calculated scheme for pricing and marketing
its Hepatitis C drug..."
United States Senate Committee on Finance, "Wyden-Grassley
Sovaldi Investigation Finds Revenue-Driven Pricing Strategy
Behind $84,000 Hepatitis Drug," press release, December 1,
2015, http://www.finance.senate.gov/ranking-members-news/
wyden-grassley-sovaldi-investigation-finds-revenue-driven-
pricing-strategy-behind-84-000-hepatitis-drug.
The full text of the 134-page report can be found at http://www.
finance.senate.gov/imo/media/doc/1%20The%20Price%20of%20
sovaldi%20and%20Its%20Impact%20on%20the%20U.S.%20
Health%20Care%20System%20(Full%20Report).pdf.